Personal P★litical Power

NAVENA

For Physicians
And Medical Practice Managers

Joel Blackwell

The Grass Roots Guy

www.PersonalPoliticalPower.com

2020 Pennsylvania Avenue NW #929

Washington DC 20006

202.277.5209

GrassRootsGuy@PersonalPoliticalPower.com

Published in the United States Of America

© 2009 by Joel Blackwell

Library of Congress Cataloging-in-Publication Data

Blackwell, Joel, 1944–

Personal Political Power For Physicians
And Medical Practice Managers / Joel Blackwell

ISBN: 978-0-9669236-2-9

1. Political Participation – United States 2. Political Activists – United States

Printed in United States of America

Contents

Part I: The Process

Part II: The People

Academics: What Scientific Research Shows About Grassroots

Lobbyists: Paid Professionals Who Usually Don't Smoke Cigars

Politicians: How Do They Want To Be Influenced?

Staff: Influential And Key To Your Success

We in America do not have government by the majority. We have government by the majority who participate.

Thomas Jefferson

You Can Join The Political Elite

In the 2004 presidential election, more than half of registered voters turned out in many places. In 2008, it was over 80%. But in most elections, particularly in primaries where most elections are decided, only 20% to 40% of Americans vote. An even smaller number makes meaningful contact with an elected officeholder about an issue during the campaign or after the election.

That so few people vote, that far fewer write or make phone calls to politicians, and almost none give money or time means that those who do communicate wield disproportionate power. People who write, make contributions and phone calls or give time to politicians form a small political elite that drives public policy.

My experience and that of many other political professionals tells me that less than 1% of Americans communicate often enough and effectively enough to influence policy. You can be in that political elite.

This book shows you how.

Introduction/Executive Summary

Personal Political Power for Physicians and Medical Practice Managers is divided into two parts. Part I gives you a proven system to maximize your influence on political legislators, state and federal. Part II contains interviews with successful volunteer advocates, paid professional lobbyists, academic researchers and politicians.

You will notice that these interviews are sometimes repetitious (everyone seems to be saying the same thing). This is important so you understand how much power you can have. If I had included a thousand more interviews, they would all have said the same thing. The message is clear: You can have incredible Personal Political Power.

The book is about getting results on political issues. It is not for what people in politics call "case work," a personal problem that affects only you. If you are trying to get some benefit like that, the staff of your elected officials will help eagerly.

Get What You Want

That's their job and they are happy to help if they can, because politicians know every successful case turns into votes. So if you aren't getting results, you probably want something you don't deserve or that is impossible to obtain. Get therapy.

Issues and policy, on the other hand, are things that might be decided by a vote in your city council, county commission, legislature or the Congress. One important operating principle: Don't expect politicians to pay attention to you if you represent just one person with a need or good idea, no matter how many people it might affect. They don't have time to devote to such matters because there are too many equally good ideas that have widespread support from broad-based organizations called special interest groups.

Am I saying you probably won't get much unless you are part of a special interest group? Yes, and rightfully so.

You will often hear politicians, even experienced ones, deriding the power of "special interest groups." The newspapers and television routinely portray them as a human version of the AIDS virus – a plague upon the Republic that needs to be eradicated. I hope when you've finished this book you have a different view. I hope you will see how the Constitution supports and enables special interest groups and what an important and positive contribution they make to our democracy. In fact, our democracy is designed and intended to foster the formation of special interest groups.

Special Interest Groups – Where It's At

Next time you hear a politician railing against "special interest groups," ask this: "Which special interest groups have too much power and what would you do to curtail it? AMA? AARP? NRA? Teachers? School boards? Realtors? Boy Scouts? Catholic Church? Insurance agents? Fact is, any honest politician will tell you that the government, and certainly the politicians, couldn't function without special interest lobbying groups with their volunteer and professional staff.

"Lobbyists are in many cases expert technicians and capable of explaining complex and difficult subjects in a clear, understandable fashion. They engage in personal discussions with Members of Congress in which they can explain in detail the reasons for positions they advocate.... Because our congressional representation is based on geographical boundaries, the lobbyists who speak for the various economic, commercial, and other functional interests of this country serve a very useful purpose and have assumed an important role in the legislative process."

Senator JOHN F. KENNEDY—Congressional Record, March 2, 1956, vol. 102, pp. 3802–3.

If you want to change law or policy in any political area – city, county, state or the United States – you need to show broad based support. You do that by forming a special interest group and mobilizing people who can vote for the politicians who can give you what you want.

The following pages explain how things work in real life. If you don't like the system, change it. On some structural issues, such as money, many politicians and lobbyists will agree with you. I probably agree with you. But for today, I'm trying to help you get what you want from the system as it exists, using tried and proven techniques.

Basic concepts you need to understand:

- Our political system is not designed to decide who is right or wrong. It is designed to decide who has a majority.

- If you can't prove that lots of people are with you, enough to get a majority of *politicians* with you, you will fail.

- There are no right or wrong positions in politics, just decisions made by human beings for good reasons or bad reasons, or out of indifference.

- If you have the votes in the legislature or Congress, you get what you want. You're right. If you don't, you get nothing. You're wrong.

- No political decision is permanent; the fat lady never sings.

I had a transformational moment years ago when I ran for office. I came to understand the most important dynamic in politics – the special relationship between politicians and the people who put them in office, the voters in their district.

Elected officials lust for voter approval. Voters are the most important people in the world, and you, as a candidate or elected official, must pay attention to them. They are your customers, and if they don't buy what you are selling, you will go out of business.

People who have been elected will always listen to the people who can vote for them, or else.

This concept became clear as I ran for the state legislature in North Carolina. I spent a lot of time shaking hands and talking with voters. Later I spoke with politicians and plumbed the vast research into how elected officials and politicians make decisions. I learned a lot about how politicians feel about the people who can vote for them.

(In case you're wondering, after a hard campaign I received many congratulations for a good race. I held my opponent to 76% of the vote.)

My goal is to get every concerned American to speak, as a representative or member of an organized group, to the people they vote for, just as the writers of the Constitution intended. If we do that, we can solve every problem the nation faces.

Are You Drowning In Cynicism?

But I fear that Americans will sink into cynicism and doubt about our political system. Our system is in danger because too many people are political dropouts. Almost everything you see on TV or read in the newspaper feeds that cynical point of view.

The presentation of politics in newspapers and television feeds negativity and gives people an easy excuse to shun political activity. The hypercritical, negative and mostly un-informed blogosphere only adds to this toxic stew. To an outsider, it all seems about money, power, and, sometimes, sex. That is not the reality I have experienced. Our system is not perfect by any stretch, but it works for those who work it. People aren't left out; they drop out.

It amazes me, as I work with ordinary people from San Diego to Boston to Miami, that those who get involved get results. They don't always get everything they want – nobody does – but they believe there is a fair process and they often win something.

Interestingly, and contrary to the image presented in newspapers and on TV, nearly all of those people who talk to politicians and work with them will tell you that elected officeholders are honest, hardworking men and women of high ethical standards who are trying their best to find satisfactory compromises to complicated problems.

Sadly, many people fall into the trap of believing that the corruption and failures reported in the media accurately represent all politicians. If you are in that group, just note that what you are seeing are the people who got caught. This proves the system usually works.

If you respond by saying, "Well, there are plenty who don't get caught," I disagree. Nobody is watched more than elected officials. It is difficult to do anything without the whole world finding out. My experience and gut feeling is that politicians are more honest than most people if for no other reason than it is so difficult for them to escape scrutiny.

Taking Money Isn't Always Corruption

It is true that many politicians operate within the cycle of taking campaign contributions, then helping those contributors achieve their goals, then getting more contributions. That's legal and doesn't mean they were bought. It's a symbiotic relationship. Note that the campaign contributions DO NOT go to the candidate but to their campaign – an important distinction.

I also believe, and this is based on conversations with hundreds of staff, politicians and lobbyists, that most people run for office out of a sincere desire to do good, as they define "good."

Whether you believe that or not, I can promise you that adopting a positive attitude is the first step toward getting what you want, while maintaining a negative attitude will do nothing but hurt you.

I hope this book will energize you to understand the constitutional role of special interest groups, become engaged and make this democracy work. We don't have political parties that engage citizens to pass legislation. As the founders intended, our system has evolved into a special interest democracy. One of my favorite clients over the years has been Realtors. They are fond of saying, "We're not Democrats; we're not Republicans. We are the Realtor Party."

We form and express consensus through myriad organizations, not political parties. That's how advocates gather the critical mass of political weight needed to move Congress or a legislature. It's very important to understand this. When you read in the newspapers or see on TV that the "Democratic Party" or the "Republican Party" has done something in Congress or a state legislature, it's misleading. A better description would be, "the Democratic caucus" or "some Republicans."

It's All About Parties, Right? Not So Fast

To call movers and shakers a "party" invokes an image of citizen participation that simply doesn't exist. We don't enact legislation through parties but through special interest groups. If you doubt this, go down to any political party office three months after an election, if you can find one. Try to "join" the party to advocate for your issue. Let me know what happens.

In my seminars I tell people, "All things being equal, politicians will go with the flow. Your job is to create the flow." You can only do that if you represent a consensus rather than a single individual. Usually this means an organization of the sort envisioned in the First Amendment: special interest groups contributing to public discourse and forming public policy.

For any bill that matters, it takes 60 votes in the U.S. Senate and 218 in the House to pass. After that, you need the support of the President and then you have to work with the bureaucrats or regulators. Those people can give you what you want.

Think of it like being in school. You can get 100% or an A in a class or you can get 70% or a C; either way, you pass. Anything less than a 70% or C grade and you don't pass. When you add 218 in the House and 60 in the Senate, you pass. Anything else is gravy. So these are the magic numbers.

(If you face a presidential veto, to override it will take a two-thirds vote in both houses: 67 in the senate and 290 in the house. Good luck!) In your state legislature, it also takes a magic number. Find out what that number is for your issue and develop your strategy. You can get what you want when you get to that number. For most issues, you can succeed with far fewer, but with those numbers, you can't lose.

The Four Essential Tools You Need

1. **Professional lobbying staff.** You need someone on the inside who understands the system and who will focus on your issues 24/7/365. A volunteer cannot devote the necessary time and can't know enough. Professional staff should help you develop a list of target politicians (who can give you what you want), develop an inside strategy, and tell you what to do and when to do it. The "inside" strategy is the plan to get votes in committee and on the floor and get a bill passed or stopped. The "outside" strategy is how to use money, media, and grassroots advocates in the district to persuade those politicians to vote with you.

2. **Money.** Anybody who is determined and has something rational to say can get a politician to listen. Just like everyone else, politicians listen best and pay the most attention to people they know and like, and who have been supportive. Money demonstrates support. Realize that while money helps, you will not be able to buy a vote in most cases. Plenty of groups win without money.

3. **Media.** Newspapers set the political agenda in their circulation area. Television doesn't. If a newspaper says an issue is important with coverage and editorials, then politicians (and television) will pay attention. Using media to amplify and deliver your message can be a powerful tool. Getting coverage on the editorial pages, in the news pages and on TV can get the attention of politicians whose help you need. For the time being, I don't see bloggers and other Internet media impacting politicians on legislative issues. That may be changing. For example, it might be that individual politicians come under much greater scrutiny on a day-to-day basis through the 'net. Whether Barack Obama's vast e-mail list, or anyone else's, can be mobilized effectively toward legislation remains to be seen.

4. **Members.** As a participant in an organization, your job is to communicate a specific message to the politician in whose district you work or vote. You must convince them that (1) a lot of people (2) in the district (3) whom the politician needs (4) care about the issue and (5) care a lot. You accomplish this by describing how the issue affects your life, your work and you and by getting others to do the same in a thoughtful, personal manner.

You have enormous power when you tell your personal story, the story of your job, your profession, your practice, your patients and the other people who can vote for the politician you are talking to. It's almost as strong even if you don't physically live in the district, but work there. ("District" refers to the area represented by U.S. House members and members of state legislatures. The "district" for U.S. Senators is their state.)

If you have a medical practice in a politician's district, they care about you. You have information valuable to them even if you don't vote there.

Politicians Need You

Again and again politicians say that they need people like you to help them understand how policy plays out in real life. What is the impact on the street? How are real people in the community affected? You are an expert on this because you live and breathe it every day.

When you realize you only have to talk about the subjects you already know, it makes your job easier. You don't have to be an expert on parliamentary procedure, the committee system or anything else. You do not need to know how a bill moves through the legislature, although that is useful. Just tell your story.

You come to your elected official as an expert in healthcare, medicine and the community. You know more than they do. You probably know more than the professional lobbyist knows. Your elected officials want to benefit from your knowledge and experience. You can also make the story come alive with personal experiences and specific stories that put a face on the issue and make it memorable.

Your ability to win in the legislature or Congress rests more on your ability to make the issue come alive with true stories than any other single factor. Every time I ask a politician to give an example of being influenced, they tell about someone who put a face on the issue with a personal anecdote. Like soap opera fans, they love a good story.

What is Grassroots Politics?

If you search the Internet for "grassroots" or "grass roots," you will get a lot of lawn companies, florists and political organizations of all kinds.

"Grassroots" in a political sense means organized at the most basic level, individual people. Rudyard Kipling used "grassroots" in his 1901 novel "Kim" to mean the origin or source ("Not till I came to Shamlegh could I meditate upon the Course of Things, or trace the running grass-roots of Evil").

In the United States, the first use of the word "grassroots" in a political sense is usually attributed to Senator Albert Jeremiah Beveridge of Indiana. He said of the Progressives Party in 1912 that "This party has come from the grass roots. It has grown from the soil of people's hard necessities."

I use the term to describe the most powerful moment in politics: constituents talking, writing, phoning and meeting with the person for whom they can vote. That's how you create Personal Political Power.

PART I
The Process

Get What You Want from Government

If you're not actually trying to solve some regulatory challenge, or fill out some form, or figure out some rule, or get the government to fund Medicare or Medicaid, at the very least you feel the hot breath of government on your neck waiting to take more of your money, or make your life difficult, or tell you where you can practice medicine, or when, or that you can't do some things at all.

Unfortunately, the government is your unwanted, incompetent business partner, one you cannot fire. Your only option is to learn how to manage it. You do that by making political action a part of your medical practice business plan and your job description. You may want to make it part of the job description of everyone in your practice.

I often ask my audiences to rate the impact and importance of government to healthcare.

Unimportant		Critical
1	_____	10

For many people, the answer is 11. That is, what government does to you or for you determines whether you thrive, survive or die. So a good question to ask yourself is: "If government is important to my practice, who is responsible for managing the government? Me or someone else? Is it in their job description? Are they rewarded for a job well done?"

Though this book is written primarily to help people in medical practice manage public policy, the same techniques will serve you well whatever your issues are.

As hard as it is to believe, you – one person – can make a difference in the course of your state and federal government.

JOEL BLACKWELL

Voting is one way, but, by far, the least powerful way. More on that later. For now, let's just say the Presidential election of 2000 delivered a wonderful wakeup call to Americans about their vote. People who failed to vote in Florida or as absentees were pulling their hair out. Then in 2004 a few changed votes in a few states would have changed the outcome.

In 2006, if you were lucky enough to live in one of the 40 or so contested House districts or six states with contested Senate races, you had a chance to change control of our government from the Republicans to the Democrats. In 2008 not only the presidential elections were hotly contested, but several senate races were decided by just a few votes. So be sure to vote.

Keep On Voting

This book is about how you can, as a practical matter, continue "voting" long after the election and have even more impact than your single vote.

This is not some dreamy, idealistic goal from a high school civics class. I see people do it all over the country. I help people do it every day in my own business.

As a consultant, trainer and speaker, I've studied, worked for and learned from the most powerful special interest groups in America – the owners and workers in real estate, banks, credit unions, nursing homes, insurance, hospitals, physician practices, law firms, colleges, farmers, oil marketers, theme parks, the NRA, AARP and unions. All the people who have clout, who get what they want from the government much of the time, are simply playing the game of politics by a set of rules.

You can do the same thing.

This book tells you how.

You can Keep On Voting and have Personal Political Power.

You already have the tools you need. The fundamentals are spelled out in the Constitution, specifically, in the First Amendment.

I'm in awe that the founding parents had the foresight more than 200 years ago to put in place a political system that would serve us so well today (I don't use "parents" to be politically correct. It took a lot of people to create this nation, and women were important though seldom recognized).

Even as recent close elections have shown, no matter what happened, there was a system in place to deal with it in a deliberate, orderly manner. How could they have looked ahead and understood the complexity of our society and given us a system that would allow everyone who chooses to participate a voice loud enough to compete?

It's a miracle.

The Source Of Power For You

I believe so much in this that on the back of my business card you will find the First Amendment – the source of your political power:

"Congress shall make no law respecting an establishment of religion, or prohibiting the free exercise thereof; or abridging the freedom of speech, or of the press; or the right of the people peaceably to assemble, and to petition the government for a redress of grievances."

Four of the five freedoms listed are yours to use to get what you want: the right to say what you think, to use that powerful megaphone we call media to amplify your voice, the right to form an organization and right to beat on the doors of your government and be heard. The fifth, religion, may even come into play: I've been known to pray for an outcome. It can't hurt.

In this book, I show you how to use your right to speak, to assemble, to petition and to use our mighty system of media to shape the healthcare system to your liking.

Tip O'Neil, Speaker of the U.S. House of Representatives, made it a famous cliché: "All politics is local." (This is also the title of his book.) Taking it a step further gave me the title "All Politics Is Personal," which is what I called my seminars for years. I wanted to use that title for this book, but it was already taken by Ralph Wright, former speaker of the Vermont House of Representatives. His book is about his political career and offers an excellent look at how legislative politics works.

The idea of politics being personal springs from the fact that all successful politicians are "people people." What they enjoy most is what Lyndon Johnson used to call "pressing the flesh." That is, getting up close and personal and dealing with real people solving real problems. Bearing this in mind, if you want to influence legislators, here's what will work:

The Top 10 Most Powerful Influencers
1. Face-to-face conversation with known constituent
2. Letter, fax or e-mail from known constituent
3. Phone call from known constituent
4. National daily newspaper article
5. National daily newspaper editorial
6. District daily newspaper article
7. District daily newspaper editorial
8. Orchestrated mail from constituents
9. Op-ed opinion pieces in major daily newspapers
10. Op-ed opinion pieces in local daily newspapers

Notice that YouTube, blogs and bloggers aren't on the list. I'm just not sure that politicians are paying attention, yet, to that vast chorus, all singing a different song. But I know these other items – even newspapers, the dinosaurs of communication – still work.

Where did this list come from? It is the result of my own research and the research done by many corporations, public affairs firms and associations.

They, and I, surveyed members of Congress and their staff to find out how they make decisions. One survey found that it takes

25 letters to influence a federal elected official who is neutral and 80 letters for one who is negative.

Not every item on this list is conclusive at any given time or in every situation. Just realize there are specific techniques to influence politicians, and among the most powerful are inputs from constituents.

The same sorts of things work on state and local elected officeholders. The results of the studies vary somewhat depending on how you ask the questions, but the basics are consistent. On most issues politicians are an open vessel, waiting to be filled. Certain techniques work to influence them. These techniques are available to you.

Other factors, such as government and academic studies and advice from bureaucrats, also have major influence. They are important because they are perceived to be objective, accurate sources. However, they are difficult or impossible for you to use because they are set up to produce objective, hard data and are often beyond influence. That just means you may have to produce your own research to counter someone else's. In my seminars, when I show the list to people, several things strike them immediately:

(1)   Constituents have a lot of power
(2)   Newspapers have a lot of power
(3)   Money isn't on the list
(4)   Voting isn't on the list

The Voting Contradiction

Some will argue that the real source of political power, for most people, is their right to vote. Certainly after the elections of 2000, 2004, 2006 and 2008, we know voting is important. In rare cases, your vote may decide who gets elected. But only rarely.

I urge my clients to get their people registered, as voting is the entry-level act to get political clout. It's important and I hope you will vote. I emphasize this because what I say next is hard for people to understand, and I want you to know that I truly believe in voting.

Voting is the least influential weapon in your political arsenal. It makes a difference by default. Bad people may get elected if you don't vote. But voting seldom creates change.

Of all our possible actions, voting is least likely to enable you to affect policy or legislation. Voting is the most difficult and costly weapon to mobilize. You can only vote every two, four or six years, and you can only vote for a few people. They may not be the ones who determine your fate. Your own member of Congress may not be in a position to help you because he or she isn't in leadership (those who control the House and Senate, the governor and president) or because they just don't have the clout.

The most your vote will do is determine who gets elected, and it only affects the district in which you live. The hotly contested presidential elections are aberrations in the context of all the elections held.

OK, Sometimes Your Vote Counts

I know, just a few votes more in Florida and Al Gore would have been president. Just a few more in Ohio and John Kerry would have been president.

Sometimes, it's close. Governor Christine Gregoire of Washington State was elected in 2004 by 129 votes out of 2.6 million cast. After the courts threw out seven votes in Montana, the Democrats gained control of the state House of Representatives. The U.S. senate race in Virginia in 2006 was very close and determined which party would be in control. Sometimes just a few votes matter. I always vote, and I hope you always do.

But in fact, outcomes of state and federal senate and house elections are rarely in doubt.

In 2004, only 31 U.S. House seats were decided by less than 10% margins. Only 20 incumbents had seriously contested races. Eighteen won, one was defeated by a challenger, one was defeated by another incumbent (Texas) after their districts were combined. In 2006, even though control of the House and Senate changed, that change was caused by voters in fewer than 40 House districts and six Senate races. Granted, if you could vote in any of those races, you really counted.

Even so, in 2006 93% of House seats did not change party hands. In the Senate it was 94%. Put another way, the incumbent or the incumbent's party was returned to office in 432 of 468 races (435 in the House and 33 in the Senate). Remember, in 2006 many people thought putting the Democrats in charge would change the course of the Iraq war.

In 2008 the Democrats increased their majority in both houses, but it remains to be seen what that will do to policy. Barack Obama quickly came under criticism from his own party for pulling back on some of his campaign promises.

Since 1996 more than 98% of incumbents have been re-elected. This is important: 98+% of people in office will stay in office as long as they want and legally can, and there is nothing you can do about it. Even if you back a candidate who wins, your person may never have significant influence and may never be a player in the issues that are important to you.

What Will Candidates Do After Elected?

Regardless of its power, our election process does not tell candidates what to do after they are elected. Because of the election process we have today, where candidates usually are selected in primaries rather than by parties, it often doesn't make a lot of difference who gets elected. The people who might win are not radically different.

Just look at presidential elections: Does the president ever turn government dramatically in one direction or another? No.

Even though his opponents may hate him for whatever reason, the fact is that we have about the same kind of government we would have had no matter who was elected on most issues. What drives public policy is less the person in office than the people pushing up from the bottom, and they change much more slowly, almost imperceptibly.

Okay, if you were on welfare during the Clinton years, maybe. If you were a member of the armed services and didn't want to go to Iraq, maybe. If you were a privacy advocate during the Bush years, okay. If you oppose torture techniques on terrorists, then fine.

But the other 99% of issues before the country? Little or no difference. What about the great Republican revolution of 1994? Did it change your life? Even the Contract for America – which mostly passed in the House of Representatives – resulted in only a few minor changes.

Did you notice how the government downsized and the budget was reduced and balanced after the Republicans controlled the House, the Senate and the White House?

Did you notice how President Obama immediately postponed or backpedaled on things he had said during the campaign. You might think you would get dramatically different results from John McCain or Ralph Nader or George W. Bush. Not really. Yes, there are areas where they differ significantly. And on a few hot button issues, McCain might have been dramatically different from Obama.

It's The Strongest Push That Counts

On most of your issues in the practice of medicine, senators, representatives and the President will go with the strongest flow. The major factor is how well you demonstrate that you have more political support than your opponents and how well you present your issue. The competition is less between parties and philosophies than it is among all the issues competing for attention.

This is the good news!

Don't be discouraged. It doesn't mean that they can't or won't help you. It doesn't mean our system of democracy is failing. In fact, if anything, this is the root of our salvation and the reason I retain a deep and abiding faith in our democracy.

Because there is one thing politicians do care about: getting elected and re-elected. That is and should be their primary goal. Many people will say with disdain, "She only wants to get elected." Of course she does. Politicians' behavior is shaped by a desire to be elected. That gives you power.

You see, although they may not know or care about your issues, you can get them to care about you, especially when you live or work in their district and are therefore a constituent. You are one of theirs if you work in a medical practice or hospital in their district or live in their district. If you work in one district and live in another, you have a twofer: two sets of politicians who can care about you.

The Most Powerful Moment In Politics

The most powerful moment in politics is when a voter talks with the person for whom they can vote. It's true during the campaign. It's true after they win. Members of the U.S. House and many state legislatures run for office every two years. That means they are always looking over their shoulder for someone who might run against them and are looking ahead for voters in the next election.

It is hard to understand this if you have not run for office. But I can tell you that someone who is campaigning will give his or her full attention to a voter. If you can vote for me, you will have my undivided attention.

In a politician's mind, you can do something most professional lobbyists cannot do and no special interest group can do: You can vote for me. I not only want your vote, I lust for it, and just as important, the approval it represents.

I have asked hundreds of state and federal elected officials across the country and they all confirm this effect. When running for or serving in office, you lust not only for contact but also for approval. Your eyes are always on the next election, and any voter who gets irritated could start a ripple across the district. (U.S. senators are a possible exception, since they only run every six years. But even they must keep a wary eye over their shoulder, especially in the two years before an election.)

You may be wondering how I can say this and say that casting your vote is the least important weapon in your political arsenal.

In most cases your vote really isn't going to make a difference, unless you and many others don't vote. I'm sorry, but your vote is probably very predictable just as is mine and everybody else's. You've heard of the red states and the blue states and red districts and blue districts. They are predictably Republican or Democratic. Most U.S. House districts and state house and senate districts are predictable because they have been designed to re-elect the incumbent, or someone just like them. In presidential and governor elections, the election will be decided by the 5 percent or so of swing voters, those who vote for a Democrat sometimes, a Republican sometimes, or even an independent.

They May Never Care About Your Issue

But it is the lust of elected officials for election and for approval by voters – all voters – that is your most important weapon. They don't know how you voted. They don't know how anyone is going to vote. All they know is that they have to try to convert every person they meet into a supporter.

It would be difficult to overstate the urgent drive in a politician to win support, love and admiration from every person who can cast a vote.

Face it: candidates and elected officials may never know or care about your issues. Your best option is to make them care about you and what you can do to elect them. Then they may care about your issues.

In the following pages, I'll show you how smart individuals and organizations do it, emphasizing three major areas: (1) attitude, (2) relationship and (3) message. You'll notice one thing is missing: that chart you may have seen titled "How a Bill Moves through the Legislature." I don't care if you don't know how that works. Don't waste your time trying to learn the process. I'll tell you how to get around that.

More important is the principle that you are going to build the right kind of long-term relationship with the people you can vote for. Then use that relationship under the direction of people in your association who really know "how a bill moves through the legislature." Let them tell you what to do and when to do it, and you will be all right.

A Reflection On A Simple Technique

As I was closing a seminar in Washington once, a woman stood up to get my attention. She was obviously very agitated. I thought she was angry. "Joel," she shouted, "you left something out." She went on to explain that she had been in my seminar the year before and I said something that changed her life.

"You told us last year that the people who write the letters, write the laws. I took it to heart and went home and started writing letters, and it's true. They pay attention." The audience applauded. All I could do was thank her.

I appreciated the endorsement, and it sounds like something I would say because I believe it. But to be honest, I did not remember saying that, although I have many times since.

Attitude:
Get Your Mind in the Right Place

In politics, as in the rest of your life, attitude can hurt or help you. When I start working with a group of people who want to win in politics, one of the first things I do is play a word association game. I ask them to give me the first word that pops into their mind when I say "politics." When a group responds with "sleaze," "crooked," "selfish," "greed," and other negative words, then I know I am speaking to people with very little political experience.

Other groups, often those who are most successful at getting what they want from the government, respond with words like "caring," "sincere," "dedicated," "hardworking," and "honest." Two things become obvious immediately: (1) people with little experience in politics have a negative image of politics and (2) most people who participate in the system have a positive image.

Why is that? How is it that the people who are in direct contact feel good, and the ones out of touch feel bad? How can they feel so bad about something they have no direct experience with?

After hearing this enough, I started asking focus groups questions such as, "Since you really haven't been involved, what causes you to form this opinion about politics?" The answer always came back loud and clear: the media. People who feel negative about politics have accepted what they read in the newspapers and see on television.

In case you have negative feelings about politics and politicians, let me offer a few thoughts. Consider the things you know about – your practice, the profession of medicine, your hospitals. Does the media do a good job of reporting on these things? Do they give a thorough, complete and accurate report?

If you only read the newspapers and watched TV, would you have an accurate impression about any of these?

Unless you're highly unusual, the answer is "Absolutely not." That's because the media report on the exceptional, the unusual, the entertaining, the failures. The media folks, and I used to be one, look for controversy, conflict and contention.

It doesn't meet their definition of news to report that a member of Congress or the state legislature works hard, serves the district well, listens to the constituents and tries to make rational sense out of a lot of complex problems. It's not news that a member of your legislature is honest.

The news you get about politics is like much of the news you get about everything else – the exceptional, which in the news media means the failures. What you have constantly hammered into your consciousness are the failures of our political system and the healthcare system.

Campaigns Are Just A Small Part Of Politics

But there's another even more important effect that contributes to the negativity many people feel about politics. Much of what is reported about politics is about campaigns. As soon as one is over they start speculating about the next one. Campaigns are by nature contentious, adversarial, controversial. The story is scripted to focus on conflict. This is called the horse race story: who's up, who's down, who's ahead, who scored, who didn't.

If you are campaigning, the name of the game is to slam your opponent.

It's like football. It's a contact sport. It's rough and people get hurt. I don't mean to defend negative campaigning. But it is important to recognize that it is campaigning – and media coverage of it – that largely creates the negative perception about all politics. Don't forget, campaigns have little or nothing to do with most issues that you and I care about. In fact, campaigns have very little to do with what government does. Just think about the things the Democratic and Republican candidates said about each other in the 2008 primaries.

As soon as the election was decided, little of it mattered.

Don't get me wrong…campaigns are important. Voting is important.

But campaigns and voting only decide which men and women will serve in office. Very few issues are decided in elections.

Campaigns and elections are not what we are talking about. What we are talking about – lobbying by grassroots volunteers – is what happens between the elections, after you vote. Grassroots lobbying has almost nothing to do with the things you see on TV or read in the newspapers.

Grassroots lobbying is a civilized, orderly, businesslike transaction without drama.

What Works Is Boring And Mostly Invisible

That's why you don't read about it or see it on TV. It may seem dull, but it gets things done. Believe me, it will feel much more like your day-to-day medical practice. And it should because it is part of your work.

When you vote on Election Day, that's like the day you decide who gets hired, or really, who gets elected. The next day, your mostly unlearned, unskilled new employees (your senators or representatives) report to work. Their success is determined by what happens in the ensuing weeks and months after being hired.

Just like a new employee, you need to give your newly elected officials constant direction and coaching. Just getting elected does not mean the voters, or anybody else, has told them what to do, despite comments about "the voters have spoken" or "the voters have given me a mandate."

Think of it this way: Barack Obama got 53% of the vote, so 47% didn't want him. Hardly a mandate.

Even if they do have any kind of "mandate" it will only be one issue, and that's probably not your issue. You still have to tell them what you want. If you don't, you leave them free to do whatever they choose. More significant, they will undoubtedly be hearing from people on the other side of your issues, and if they don't hear from you, you give them permission to go the other way.

Your Attitude About Advocacy

In my research into why people don't contact elected officials, one comment came up frequently: "Elected officials are too busy doing important work to talk with me." It's true they are busy. But nothing is more important to an elected official than a constituent. Just think, who puts her in office? Who is going to determine if she stays in office? You and others like you who vote in the district.

I did a grassroots training session in New York State a while back. Then I went with one of the trainees over to the Capitol to meet with her senator. When we got there, we met with a staffer who said the senator would be back shortly; he was in a meeting.

The senator was Ronald B. Stafford, chairman of the Senate Finance Committee. He eventually served 37 years before retiring and was in no danger of losing his seat. When I met him, he had been holding an important budget hearing, yet he left the meeting to come talk with this one woman from the district.

When it was over, I asked him why he left an important meeting to speak with just one voter. Here is what he said: "Because I know that anytime I don't meet with her or any of my constituents, they are going to go back home and get on the phone and call everyone they know and tell them that I'm getting too big for my britches and I have no time for someone back home. And the next election, they may send me back home."

Elected officials know, and they constantly keep in mind, who sent them to the capitol and who can send them home.

Many people think politicians don't want to hear what they have to say because the politicians have already made up their minds. On some issues, it's true; you can't change their minds. Elected officials, just like you and I, have some attitudes they will not change. I call these quasi-religious beliefs. They are deeply seated matters of faith and belief, and almost no amount of logic or persuasion will change a person's belief system.

Abortion, gun control, the death penalty – you are unlikely to change anyone's mind on those sorts of issues. Many times, not even the threat of losing an election can change a politician's mind about these issues; they would rather lose than change.

But the medical and regulatory issues you will be lobbying about are more technical and invisible to most elected officials, most voters and the media. They are less a matter of faith than of practicality. You are concerned about reimbursement, access and insurance. This sort of issue is not likely to be discussed in depth in a campaign and isn't likely to become an important part of a campaign.

Your elected official probably knows little or nothing about reimbursement. They don't have to do coding or file insurance claims, so they are waiting to be informed and persuaded. These are the 99.44% of issues that take up time in state legislatures and the Congress. Any of them could probably be decided any way and the Republic would survive just fine.

Politicians, For The Most Part, Just Don't Care

This is true of most medical issues. History is unlikely to change regardless of which way your senator or representative votes. Politicians are willing to listen to any sensible suggestion for a change. They have no emotional or political stake to defend and are willing to be persuaded.

Remember, since most issues of medicine never come up in a campaign and they haven't learned about them some other way, elected officials go into office as empty vessels—they don't know your issue and they don't care. They can vote whichever way the wind is blowing or whichever way someone nudges them. Somebody is going to help them decide what they think. It can be you, particularly if you live or work in their district. You can create or change their opinion.

But first, you have to persuade them to care at all. If you can convince them that enough voters in their district or enough important and well-informed people in the district care, then they will care. Then you have a chance to persuade them to support your position. That's a main source of power for you. (I will explain how you can become important to your elected official when we get to relationship building.)

You can make a difference because you vote in their district or work in their district and have contacts there. They care about you and what you think, even if they don't know or care about your issue. Elected officials want you to go home and brag to everyone that you talked to them and they listened to what you had to say.

Even people who belong to medical or practice management associations often fail to realize their own power.

Sometimes they think they don't need to work for themselves because they have a paid professional lobbyist to do the work.

You Can Have More Power Than Lobbyists

You need that professional, the one I call the "inside lobbyist." But that lobbyist cannot vote except in one district. The professional has the power of knowledge, persuasion, personal relationship, good information and maybe fund-raising...and that's significant. But the importance of the professional lobbyist pales in comparison to someone who lives and votes or works in the district.

Look at it from the standpoint of an elected official. Imagine that I am your senator. I may like your professional lobbyist. I may respect the lobbyist. But she needs me more than I need her. I can accept her information, reject it or just ignore it. If I kiss off or ignore your lobbyist, so what? That lobbyist can hardly try to get even with me for fear that I will remember it the next time she needs me.

But as your senator, when someone who can vote for me says people in my district care about an issue, I have to listen if I want to stay in office.

I can't afford to have people back home saying negative things about me. You are a substantial member of my community and not only do I want you saying positive things about me, I really don't want you saying negative things.

What's more, you can help me understand why something is important in my district. After all, I want to represent that district.

Worried About The Risk Of Involvement?

Perhaps you don't advocate for your issues because you are worried about getting into controversy and somehow someone will retaliate. You are concerned that something bad will happen as a result.

It's just not likely.

Think about the issues you are discussing. Reimbursement, scope of practice, funding for education, liability, electronic medical records. These issues are not like abortion or gun control, where everybody has an opinion and strong feelings.

Most medical issues are not the kind of thing anyone will get emotional about. No one except you and your opponents care. Most issues never even make the back section of the newspaper, much less the television.

As long as you stick to issues and avoid personal references, it's hard to imagine any negative result. Even the most nonpartisan, apolitical group is expected to advocate or educate to win support for its goals. Politicians want and need your expertise and experience. Recognize the difference between supporting issues and candidates. As long as you stick to your issues and skip personalities and endorsing candidates, you will stay out of trouble.

Despite media reports to the contrary, Americans are usually able to disagree agreeably. The traditional media folks have to emphasize conflict and maximize the appearance of conflict or they lose their audience. The bloggers, shout TV and talk radio are even worse. Do not accept their portrayal of politics as reality.

Another obstacle to advocacy is time. We're all so busy surviving, dealing with family and jobs; we think we don't have time to get involved in politics. You may envision "getting involved" as having to stay on the phone, go to a lot of meetings, write a lot of letters, and travel to the Capitol.

Not so.

If you are focused on one issue, you probably won't need to write or call more than six times as the legislation moves through the process. If you make contact six times, taking less than a half hour each time, you can have significant impact. How long does it take to scribble a note and fax it or to make a phone call urging support?

The Most Powerful System You Can Use

Most of the organizations you would say have political clout get it by using what is generically called a "key contact" system.

A Key Contact is a person who volunteers to build a relationship with a specific politician and carry the message from the practice or association to that politician.

As a key contact, you would be very busy if you were asked to contact your elected official more than ten times in a year. That means unless things are really hopping, you might be asked to make ten phone calls or write ten letters. That's it. Figuring a maximum of one-half hour each, you have invested five hours.

Most key contacts write fewer than four letters and make fewer than four calls or personal contacts. Even if you double or triple it, you aren't risking overload. Aren't you willing to commit five to fifteen hours in the next twelve months to achieve the political goals necessary for a successful practice?

If everyone who has a stake in your medical group would commit those few hours, you would be unstoppable. You would have an unbeatable political machine. That's without even leaving your office. As for going to the Capitol, it can be useful and fun, but it's not necessary.

In fact, when you become a volunteer advocate for your association, your best work is done at home in the district. You drink coffee with your elected official, you attend meetings, you invite the politicians to come into your practice or hospital and you represent your association in the district. These contacts are much more powerful coming from constituents in the home district. They don't take much time or travel and lots of good work is accomplished during times and in places that you are doing other things anyway.

Your Attitude About The Buildings

As we researched the reasons average citizens don't get involved in lobbying, one answer came up time and time again that surprised me. "The buildings intimidate me."

I chuckled the first time I heard this. But then as my focus group work proceeded, it became obvious – the buildings are a factor in alienating people. Of course, as I said, you don't have to go to the Capitol or other government buildings. But there are times when it's useful. You will find it's fun.

But to get over that intimidation factor I started asking the question, "What is it about the buildings?" Finally it came to me: Our capitol buildings were designed to intimidate. The United States Capitol and many state capitols are modeled after Greek and

Roman architecture in neoclassical style. Those Greeks and Romans weren't building malls designed to attract lots of people. They were building temples to the gods. They were designed to inspire awe and to intimidate ordinary people.

Picture the standard capitol. It is usually on a hill, often the highest ground for miles. You walk through meticulously groomed park like grounds, up a long flight of stairs, through tall stone columns, huge doors and metal detectors. You're scrutinized by short-haired muscular people in uniforms with guns, and then walk into elaborately decorated high-ceilinged rooms.

(If you live in New Jersey, this does not apply. It's intimidating, but mostly because it looks like a haven for muggers. In Lincoln, Neb., where everything is flat, there was no high ground to use. But they did the best they could. The statue of a boy sowing wheat seeds on top of the capitol is the highest point in the Great Plains. In New Mexico, they call the capitol the roundhouse. It is. But I digress.)

Who wouldn't be intimidated? One woman told me she walked into the capitol in Albany, New York, and had to fight off the impulse to kneel and genuflect. She felt as though she had walked into a cathedral. It's easy to be overwhelmed by the hustle and bustle and confusion. I still get lost almost every time I take a group of volunteer lobbyists to the office buildings in Washington.

So if it's any help, most of us who don't work there every day are in awe of the buildings. The answer is to barge on in, understanding that those are your buildings; you bought and paid for them. When you get in, you will find a lot of friendly people who will help you because they all know the buildings are yours. It won't take long to overcome your fear.

Your Attitude About Yourself

Many people say to me, "I'm afraid to talk to a member of Congress. I don't know what to say."

Yes, you do. In your field you are the expert. You are the frontline trooper dealing with it every day. You see and live with the results of legislation.

Many elected officials know nothing about business in general, healthcare or medicine in particular. But they want to. Many of them come out of law. Some were journalists. Some have been Realtors. Some were homemakers.

Whatever they were, they won't know about your practice and needs unless you tell them. You can be confident you know more than your senator or representative about the practice of medicine and your community through your patients. You know how you are affected and how others are affected. And that's all you need to talk to them about – your daily experience.

This is particularly true for those elected officials who go to Washington and live in an increasingly isolated Never Never Land. They know it. When you ask them, as I have, they always say the one thing they miss most is the day-to-day contact with real people who can express the real needs of the community. You can fill that void. Your elected official wants to hear from you, and you have valuable information to give them.

Your Attitude About Your Rights

Think for a moment about this question: Where do you get the right to lobby? We seem to be a nation of complainers. We take it for granted that we have the right to blame the government for everything and to try to get the government to fix everything.

But step back and think about it for a moment. Where do you get the right to lobby? Most people eventually answer, "It's in the Constitution."

Of course. After thinking for a while, you might have said it is in the Bill of Rights, perhaps freedom of speech. Although you are close, it's more specific than that. Remember the First Amendment to the Constitution:

*Congress shall make no law respecting an
establishment of religion, or prohibiting the free
exercise thereof; or abridging the freedom of speech,
or of the press; or the right of the people peaceably to
assemble and to petition the government for a redress
of grievances.*

Your right to lobby is spelled out in the First Amendment: "to
petition the government for a redress of grievances."

Do you remember from history class how the Bill of Rights –
the First Ten Amendments – came to be written? Our ancestors
had just come through a long and bloody war (about eight years)
and had created the Articles of Confederation to bring the states
together. That didn't work, so they came back and wrote the
Constitution. But some states wouldn't sign until they added the
Bill of Rights, including the First Amendment.

You Have All The Tools You Need

In that First Amendment, they spelled out your most important
rights. It's obvious, given what they had been through, that
religion, press, assembly and speech would merit protection. But
why did they put your right to lobby in the First Amendment with
freedom of religion, speech, press and assembly? Because they
had not had that right.

Historically, the king in England ruled by divine right and
could not be questioned. The citizens did not have the right to
petition for a redress of grievances.

Your ancestors understood that only if the people had the
right to complain – constantly – would government have to
listen and respond.

This right is one of the founding principles of democracy that separates us from a lot of the rest of the world. This is one reason people from around the world want to come here. It is one reason why I urge you to make lobbying a part of your personal and professional plans and goals.

It is important to understand your key role in making this democracy work by exercising your right to complain. I would even go further. You not only have the right to lobby, but it is your obligation, your responsibility.

It's important for you to let your government know what you want and don't want. It's a way of repaying those people who, two hundred years ago, gave us everything we have today.

It's a way of making sure that those who come behind us enjoy the same privileges we do. When you work through your association on behalf of your practice, your patients and yourself, you are not only working for that narrow interest, but you are also making this democracy work the way the founding parents envisioned it.

As I said in the introduction, one of my goals in life is to get all Americans to contact the people they vote for. I am convinced if we can do that, we can solve every problem that faces us. Though I may not be able to get every single American energized enough to write or make a phone call, I hope you will. I hope you will become one of those people who make democracy work.

It all starts with your attitude about politics, politicians and yourself.

Associations: Special Interest Groups Make It Happen

You can have a powerful influence over elected officials, particularly when you are talking to the ones you can vote for. But no politician would or should act just because you, or any other one person, have a great idea.

They won't because, if they are experienced, they know they only have a certain amount of political capital to spend. They won't waste it on causes they can't win.

Remember the "magic numbers" from earlier? John McGoughlin, a state representative in North Carolina, explained it this way: "There are lots of good ideas out there. Really good ideas. They are practical. They will work. They will accomplish some useful social goal. But they don't have the political support to go anywhere. At every step in the process you must have 50% plus one or you die."

A nice dose of realism. It doesn't matter how righteous your cause is. If you can't show widespread support, your issue will die. And it should. Politics is the art of finding the middle, building consensus and then creating a majority. One person's idea, no matter how good it is, will not and should not be given serious consideration just because it's a good idea.

Only those ideas that have, or reasonably might have, or someone can cause to have, widespread support are worthy of becoming public policy. Setting majority rule and democracy aside, ideas without widespread support will not work.

It Takes An Organization

The way you demonstrate widespread support is through an organization.

Most often political goals are achieved through an association of people, either formal or informal (as in a coalition). If you don't represent something larger than yourself and your good idea, you are unlikely to be taken seriously.

It's like a newspaper op-ed page (that's the page across from or opposite the editorials with columns and articles of opinion). I could submit an article outlining a brilliant public health initiative to combat teenage pregnancy. I might get it published as a brief letter to the editor. It wouldn't merit anything more because what I think on that topic, no matter how good the idea, isn't worth much.

If the surgeon general or the chair of a senate committee wrote an identical article, it could get major play around the country. It would be taken seriously because it would represent some significant constituency, something larger than one person's good idea.

For purposes of this book, we assume that you are a member of an association. (If you aren't, join one now or never complain again.) This usually provides you with the next essential ingredient: the professional lobbyist.

You must have someone on the inside who understands the players and the process and who can lead you through the minefield of legislative deliberation. Think of it in terms of a sports metaphor: the association members are the team. They carry the ball and they score. The professional lobbyist is your coach, providing the experience and judgment to bring your talent and energy to bear in the right place at the right time.

"Professional adviser" usually means a paid lobbyist who is working for you. But I have seen instances where volunteer advocates had the time and knowledge to do the job well. Another possibility is your own elected official. If you can get her interested in your issue, she may be able to help you chart a course through the legislature or Congress.

Pros Do Something You Can't Do

The keys to success for most associations are (1) get a professional lobbyist and (2) obey them. Unless you are focused on politics and your issue 24/7/365, understand the system, know the major players and personalities and understand their motivations, and have the commitment and time to focus virtually all your energy on the political system, you will make costly mistakes. It will take you too long to learn. You may never figure out how to make something happen.

The first time I tried to get some legislation passed was back in the early 1970s, when open meetings and records were a much bigger issue than they are today. Working with Common Cause, a group of us in Atlanta were trying to get the legislature to open the budget process. Our state representative, Sidney Marcus, had agreed to help us.

At one point, he told us to pull back because the Speaker of the House didn't want this legislation introduced. Sidney said he wouldn't introduce it. Since we knew the cause was just and right, we decided to pressure Sidney. We started calling him, as his constituents. We decided if we could make his phone ring often enough, we could change his mind. After one or two phone calls, he took his phone off the hook. He didn't want to deal with a bunch of fools, particularly when so many were not even from his district.

Frustrated, we found a freshman representative who agreed to introduce our bill. After he introduced it, in defiance of the Speaker of the House, the freshman got squashed and stripped of influence. Sidney, on the other hand, became chairman of a powerful committee.

Later he gave us a lot of help and advice. Because of his position, he was able to help get a lot of our ideas passed into law. Unlike us amateurs, he had enough sense and experience to know what to do and when to do it to get something done. Because we did not factor in Sidney's experience and judgment, we were left holding our ideals, knowing we had gone after the right thing, yet had gotten nothing.

Be smart. Get a professional lobbyist and follow their directions.

In and Out

I draw a distinction between what I call the "inside" (professional) lobbyist and the "outside" (volunteer) lobbyist. You need both.

The inside lobbyist is your professional legislative representative. This person knows the ins and outs of the legislature or Congress. He knows the committee system. He knows the players. He knows the arcane parliamentary rules. He knows the secret handshake and the password to get behind closed doors. He could draw a chart showing how a bill moves through the legislature in the dark. It's vital to have a person like this on your side.

But you, the volunteer advocate, the outside lobbyist, don't need any of that. Your skills and value lie in your ability to communicate to the person you vote for – to relate your personal experience and your knowledge of how things work in your practice and life back in the district at home.

Professionals provide technical details. They write and edit legislation. They discuss the broad scope and sweep of politics across a nation or state. They use logic, statistics and politics to persuade. They make the case in general. They develop strategy.

Elected officials want to know three things from you: (1) How an issue affects the people back home, (2) how much the people back home care, and (3) who cares. The bottom line is, no matter how worthy your cause, your elected official wants to know how many people care, how much do they care, and how many live in my district.

This is information that you can provide better and with more credibility than the professional lobbyist. You work and live with the people in the district; the professional lobbyist doesn't. You have a critical role in communicating your perspective as an expert in your field who lives in the district.

Know The Political Cycle Of Seasons

All professional lobbyists with whom I have talked (hundreds of them) acknowledge this effect. They will tell you that they can be much more powerful if they have a constituent with them. Much of their power derives from whatever perception the elected official has of the lobbyist's constituency.

There is something else that the professionals can do much better than we volunteer advocates: plan the strategy. They know how to work through the maze. They know about timing and when to compromise, so leave that to them.

I suggest that every organization develop strategies for four time frames that fit within political cycles. Legislative sessions are like tides; they roll in and out very predictably and determine where you put your umbrella and cooler on the beach. Depending on where you are in the cycle, think about:

1. From now until Election Day. What are you going to do in the weeks and months leading up to elections? Depending on your organization's culture, it may range from nothing to running candidates. Just make sure you have considered the election process and have a strategy. This could be a period as long as a year leading up to Election Day.

2. From Election Day until the start of the legislative session or Congress. This is when some of your best work can be done. Establish relationships with the newly elected. Strengthen relationships with those re-elected. Lay groundwork for your legislative program. Identify key decision makers and legislative gatekeepers. Test your volunteers to see who will deliver.

3. From start of session to end. What will you do in the district? Will you bring people to the Capitol? What sort of communications system will you use? What's your media strategy? What is the role of your volunteer

advocates? Do you have key contacts in targeted districts trained and ready to respond to action alerts? In states that have year-round legislatures, you must have a year-round organization.

4. The long haul. It will take years to get what you want, meaning that the immediate success or failure you achieve is not final. You and all with you must be prepared to stick with your issues through defeat and after victory. You must demonstrate a commitment strong enough to convince those in power that you are never going away.

Relationship Is Everything

I assume that you're working with others in an association and you want to have an impact on your government.

You will be better off if you realize that your primary job is building relationships. Issues come and go; you win some and lose some. But the relationships you build will serve you for a long time, win or lose.

First, realize that most elected officials run for office out of a genuine desire to serve the district they will represent. Even if they run to promote their own agenda or advocate their own issues, they soon learn that unless they are winning friends with service, they won't be in office long. So their driving impulse is to help you if they can. All things being equal, elected officials will try to help you because that's how they get re-elected and because that's why they are in office.

The problem is that they can't help all the people who want it. They must carefully choose which issues they get behind to push. A member of Congress told me once that voters have to understand, "We're here to represent you, not advocate for you."

A state legislature might see 5,000 bills introduced in an average year. Anywhere from several hundred to several thousand pass into law. The average representative or senator cannot give careful consideration to more than a handful. She cannot lead the charge on more than one or two.

How does she choose? How can you get her to choose to represent your issue? Look at what an elected official's priorities will be on issues:

First, she will try to push the things she believes in, the things that were important in her campaign. Most of those will fall by the wayside because they have no support. Issues that win elections often have a hard time finding their way into law. (Your issues are unlikely to have been part of any campaign.)

Second, she will support issues important to leadership. Those who control the house and senate, the governor and president all have their own agenda. Your elected official, the one you vote for, has to work with them to accomplish anything.

It was that consummate legislator, Lyndon Johnson, who said, "If you want to get along, you have to go along." Most legislators, certainly those who are going anywhere, will back leadership because it makes the decision easy. The issues that leadership is backing don't take much time, either. One strategy is for you, your association, and your medical facility to get leadership to adopt your issue. This makes for easy sailing but is difficult to make happen.

The third set of issues your legislator will push is in an area where the volunteer advocate plays a key role. These issues are the ones her friends and supporters are interested in that have potential to be passed into law.

An elected official's circle of friends and supporters become her binoculars on the world. They are the filter through which the official sends and receives information and through which she views the world. It's natural enough and we all do it. How much time do you spend listening to people you don't like, don't know or don't agree with?

Build The Relationship

No matter how hard we try, we all tend to associate with people who are supportive of us and our goals. We tend to reject or screen out our opponents. We tend to ignore people we don't know in favor of those we do.

Your challenge is to get into that third set of priorities – friends and supporters. Through your association, you can get enough other people who are friends and supporters of enough other elected officials to get to the critical 50% plus one.

Remember: Your elected official probably doesn't know anything or care anything about your issue. It may be new or maybe something she puts on the way back burner. But if she knows you and cares about you, then she will allocate time and energy to help you. That's what relationship building is all about.

A key question in determining your political success is, "How can you get your elected official to care about you?" The answer will come as you consider these two questions: (1) What are her personal and political goals? (2) What have you done to help her achieve her goals?

Follow this rule: Never ask a politician for anything until you have helped her enough that she will welcome an opportunity to repay you. If you have done nothing for her, why would she help you, given that she has limited time and there are others with equally worthy goals who have already helped her? What goals of hers might you help get accomplished?

Of course, her first goal is to get re-elected. Others might be (1) to pass legislation, either a particular piece or just any bill; (2) achieve recognition: she wants people to know what she has accomplished; (3) advance to a higher political office or to more power in the current office; (4) find new problems to solve; (5) raise money (see re-election).

Each elected official will have a different set of goals. Your job, as a volunteer advocate, is to figure out what they want and help them get it.

Stand Out

You will stand out immediately from the many people who want something from a politician if you just ask, "What are your goals and how can I help you attain them?" The big number one is re-election. Have you volunteered to work in a campaign? Have you contributed significant money to your PAC (Political Action Committee) or to the election campaign?

If so, you will have access and a warm welcome. But notice, I asked, "Have you contributed significantly?" People frequently ask me how much to give. My rule of thumb is, you want to be in the top tier of contributors. You want your contribution to stand out, whether it is from a PAC or from you personally. This is another reason why PACs work.

They bring together amounts of money that will be remembered.

Contributions are a matter of public record, so find out what others are giving and give enough to stand out. People often tell me they don't feel good about giving campaign contributions. It feels like they are trying to buy a vote. Don't worry. That doesn't happen with legal campaign contributions.

For one thing, there are usually limits as to how much you can give. Also, these contributions are on the record and are usually reported in the media.

Are Your Opponents Giving To Your Guy?

It frequently happens that your opponents, the people on the other side of your issue, are also giving to the same candidate, so the money from opposing sides balances out. Obviously you are giving to promote your cause or interest. So what do you get for the money?

The best reason to give is that you may actually help elect someone who agrees with you. Presumably you are supporting your friends and opposing your enemies. The money you give to a campaign is used to pay for advertising, direct mail, phone bills – the things a person needs to do to get elected.

One politician pointed out to me, "You're not giving the money to me; you're giving it to the campaign." It's a good place to start; get "good people" (those who agree with you) in office. It's also true that you cannot expect anyone to be in 100% agreement with you 100% of the time. Just because you help elect someone does not mean she will always be with you.

However, given that most issues could go either way and the Republic would survive, and given that most politicians don't know or care about most issues, and given that their basic impulse is to help their friends and supporters, it follows that if you are a significant contributor (either by giving time or money) you get more than access. You get a warm, helping welcome.

I still believe that any citizen with something sensible to say can get a conversation with an elected official, although it may not be easy. It is in the politician's interest to at least listen. (U.S. senators from large states are the exception. Hardly anyone gets to them; they just don't have the time. Getting to their staffers is the key.)

Pitch In

But you want more. You want a relationship with your elected official that moves from professional courtesy to friendly support. You want her wanting to say yes, eager to help. Money isn't the only way.

For example, volunteering time to work in a campaign or work on a task force can be even more valuable. This may be hard to believe because of the way television and newspapers portray campaigns. When you see campaigns on television, you usually see the big national races or hotly contested races for the U.S. House or Senate. You see a carefully created picture of crowds of enthusiastic volunteers.

The reality, particularly at the state and local level, is different. The number of consistent volunteers, not paid staff, working in campaigns is very small, usually not even ten in a state race and twenty to thirty in a federal race. One state senator in Michigan told me she had to hire temps, not because she had no supporters but because they were all two-worker families with children and had no time.

You can become a valuable resource just by showing up. Think about the volunteers in Florida who completed the absentee ballot applications for the Republican Party. Think about the people who demonstrated in front of the ballot count in Miami and apparently contributed to getting the count stopped. Think about the vast cadre of Obama supporters recruited online to make phone calls at a cell phone party.

A small effort by you can make a big difference and will be remembered. You can establish a relationship and you can earn that warm, friendly access by putting out signs, making phone calls and stuffing envelopes. You can, with relatively little time investment, get on a first-name basis with your elected officials or top tier staff.

It helps to develop a specialty – something you like doing and can do well – that's valuable to a campaign. For example, if you are friendly with numbers and detail, learn how to keep track of campaign contributions and expenses. It's not hard or complicated; it just requires a good eye for detail and a lot of discipline. People who can do this are worth their weight in gold to the campaign and the candidate.

Sign Expertise Opens The Door

My specialty is signs. When I support candidates, I load up my car with signs. I pull out my special mallet (named Edna) and my heavy-duty staple gun and cruise the precincts I know best, pounding stakes and stapling signs. The mallet is named Edna after Edna Chirico, a county commissioner I supported.

I met her one day while I was out riding my bicycle. I saw her putting out signs, talked to her and asked her what I could do to help. "Put out some of these signs," she said, and I did.

Though she's no longer in office, she still remembers me. When she was in office, she would return my calls.

You can be even stronger contributing volunteers as an organization. If your association helps recruit workers, you will get that friendly access.

One group I worked with helped set up phone banks for a man running for Congress. For two weeks, they mustered between ten and twenty people every night to make calls around the district. He faced a tough fight in the primary and won by 974 votes. His name was Newt Gingrich.

Four years later he was Speaker of the House and he publicly stated that no legislation harmful to this group would pass while he was Speaker. He was as loyal to his friends as they were to him.

One easy thing to do is organize a site visit for your elected official. Let them come to your practice or hospital or to an association meeting for an appearance. If you put them in front of potential voters, put them in your newsletter or get media coverage for them, they won't forget.

Once a state senator called and asked me to write a letter to the editor. The newspaper had been covering an issue and he felt he needed to show that his side had some support. It was an issue I cared about, and I was glad to do it. It took me all of thirty minutes to write it and fax it to the newspaper. They published it. Is that senator going to answer my phone call? Will he help me if he can? You bet.

Keep Them Informed

Your elected official needs many things in addition to money and volunteer time. For example, simply knowing what's going on in the community is very important to her.

Your contacts at work, church, civic club and social relationships put you in touch with people and groups of all kinds. Think of the news you hear about a new company coming to town, a new issue some town council is discussing or something you read in a local newspaper. This may be information that doesn't make its way to your elected official. Some districts are huge, especially the congressional districts, and it's difficult for officials to keep up with what's going on.

For example, not too long ago I read in my community newspaper that a small town nearby had formed a task force on education and crowding in the elementary school. Knowing that my county commissioner probably doesn't get that paper, I faxed her a copy of the article. I wrote a note that said, "Here's a meeting you might like to know about. If you can't make it, I can attend and take notes."

She faxed me back, thanking me and saying she'd be there and hadn't known about the meeting. It took me five minutes but it was most valuable to her. She answers my phone calls and gives me a warm welcome.

This kind of activity is especially helpful in avoiding the "out of sight, out of mind" factor. To build a really good relationship, I recommend you put it on your calendar to make positive contact at least quarterly.

Stay in front of her with something that helps her so she doesn't forget. It could be as simple as a letter, a phone call or a fax, but whatever it is, do something regularly. If you see your elected official is speaking to a group, attend the meeting and shake her hand. Stand up and support her publicly.

It doesn't have to be something that advances your cause, and it's better if it doesn't. Just do something to help out or show support. Granted, this may seem simple, but it works, perhaps even more because so few people do it. Most people, if they participate in politics at all beyond complaining, vote and that's all. When you become personally engaged with your elected officials, you stand out like a warm slice of Mom's pound cake.

One Simple Step To Increase Your Power

An example of things few people do is a story about the mayor of the town where I used to live. He and I are in different political parties and we frequently disagreed. But he was a reasonable man and a hard worker. He'd been in office about ten years and had done well by our town in a job that is generally thankless.

One day we were standing out in the street, arguing about a zoning issue. Finally I said, "Okay, Russell, I can see we are never going to agree. But I would like to say one thing. I appreciate the fact that you have served in office and I want to thank you for serving. Even when we disagree, I know you have the town's best interest at heart."

He was shocked. He got a tear in his eye and said, "Joel, in the ten years I've been in office, no one has ever said that to me before." It didn't change his mind. But I'm always thinking about the next time, and he will remember what I said. You will stand out if you do nothing but thank your elected official for serving because so many people never take that one simple step.

Match Key Contacts To Politician

As I said, the mayor and I are in different political parties, and this is something that comes up often with grassroots volunteer lobbyists. Can I work well with an elected official of a different party – someone whose politics I detest? Yes and no.

Whenever possible, I recommend matching grassroots volunteers with elected officials of the same party and outlook. In the best of all worlds, the grassroots contact will be a mirror image of the elected official. But this is seldom possible. Don't worry. When you contact an elected official, she usually won't know what party you are in and won't ask. Even if you are in the other party and she knows it, your issue may not be one supported or opposed by the political parties.

In some states, Pennsylvania and Illinois for example, political party is crucial. In those states your professional adviser will tell you what to do. I do not recommend lying, but neither would I suggest you walk in and announce, "I'm in a different party." If it comes up, be honest.

Hey, I Voted For You

(Incidentally, saying you voted for her doesn't work. It sounds like you expect something in return. Oddly enough, everyone elected officials meet seems to have voted for them. I used to meet people all the time who would say they voted for me, even though they didn't live in my district.)

No matter what their party, officials know they get elected and re-elected by serving people. If they can, they want to help people in their district. It's called constituent service and they know it's what keeps them in office.

As for building a good relationship, I have found it helpful to think in terms of a "favor bank." I have an account with my elected representative just as I have one at the bank, except in this one, I deposit favors. That means you have to look for favors to do.

Analyze the person's goals and help her achieve them. You will maintain a good account balance by making regular deposits in the favor bank. Deposit the time you spent putting out signs. Deposit the time you spent stuffing envelopes. Add to your account when you contribute money.

I think of it as building up equity so I can take out a loan. Who would I like to get favors (or loans) from? In this case, I want something from elected officials. So I want to maintain a favorable balance and never overdraw my account. Before I ask for something, I want to be sure that I have built up favors that will have been remembered.

If this sounds a little too contrived, a little too cynical, remember that this is the way all friendships and relationships work. We just don't usually sit down and analyze it. We aren't methodical about maintaining the favor balance. Like it or not, it will work.

My basic rule is that there is only one time you lobby: year in, year out, year round. Never stop. Just like any relationship, there needs to be two-way giving and receiving. If that lapses, where's the relationship?

What Will You Get?

Many amateurs and newcomers think all they have to do is head off to the legislature while it's in session, make an elegant case and go home with a victory.

It never happens that easily. Politics is a long, messy process.

Another important aspect of the relationship is your expectations.

You will seldom get everything you want. You must be prepared and committed to the long haul. A major idea can easily take between five and eight years to work through.

Your political results will be in direct proportion to your ability to convey the perception that you and your organization are never going to go away. You were here last year, you were here this year and you will be here next year and the year after. Elected officials are less likely to invest serious time or effort if you do not demonstrate staying power.

There are also limits to what your elected officials can do even when they want to help you. In some legislatures and the Congress, anything that passes depends on a small cadre in leadership. You must get them behind you. There is little or nothing the elected officials who represent you can do by themselves. If leadership in the house or senate is against your issue, accept the fact that you have to convert leadership – no easy task.

Conversely, one of the great strengths of grassroots lobbying is that strong support in the district can allow your elected official to vote in your favor, even when it goes against leadership. Either opposing or not going along with leadership is dangerous. If your elected representatives are going to be effective, for you and others, they must support leadership.

Yet there are times when they don't want to as a matter of personal preference, and times when they don't want to because their constituents are on the other side of an issue. Speaker of the U.S. House of Representatives Tip O'Neil recognized this effect. When he needed to pass a bill he would often have some members who, for one reason or another, needed to vote the other way. O'Neil would sit them all in the front row. If he didn't need their votes, he would let them pass. But if he did, he expected them to vote with him. He would look them in the eye and they would know the moment had come. Can you imagine the pressure?

Going Against Leadership

So if you ask your elected official to go against leadership or to convert leadership, you have to give her a very strong reason. One powerful reason for a legislator to go against leadership, and one that leadership understands, is a strong message from the district.

This gives you power because you and your organization can provide that message. Letters, faxes, and other demonstrations of support for an issue from the district give politicians political cover, even to go against leadership.

It also means that if you live in a district represented by someone in leadership, such as the speaker or a committee chair, you have special ability to make things happen.

Timing is also important. Legislative affairs run on a schedule. Usually, by the time the session starts, the issue train is leaving the station. You need to get on that train at least six to nine months before the legislature convenes. You need to give your legislator time to absorb your information, check it out, sound out other interested parties and get back to you.

Sometimes your information needs to simmer for a while before it tastes right. You can see the importance of lobbying year in, year out and year round.

When you do talk with elected officials it is unusual, in my experience, to get a commitment. I mention this because some books advise you never to leave the presence of an elected official without a commitment. All I can say is, "Good luck." No smart, experienced elected official will ever give you a commitment until the last possible minute. That's because things can always change.

In one of my seminars, a man told me he had spoken to his representative, had a good conversation and got a firm commitment. Then the guy voted against him. When questioned about it, the representative answered, "Leadership told me to." I asked the man if this legislator was in his first term.

Yes, he was, as I expected.

An inexperienced politician may make a commitment, only to find good reasons not to keep it. But even if they have to vote against you because of leadership, all is not lost. At least now that politician owes you one.

Gauge Your Impact

As you pursue support from politicians, you may begin to see it as a sales process. Scout your prospects, qualify them, build the relationship, respond to objections and sell the benefits.

In sales, you make what is called a "trial close." That is, you check out the prospect to see how you're doing. If you can't get a commitment, you may still be able to get a sense for which way the wind is blowing by asking an open-ended, non-threatening question such as, How do you feel about what I've said so far? Is there any other information you need to make a decision? The answers will tell you what to do next.

As you work toward your goal, you will see there is a hierarchy of performance you can achieve. Volunteer lobbyists tend to move through several skill levels as they develop relationships. Let me list those for you now to help you identify your level within the big picture of volunteer lobbyists. It will help you understand more about your job and what you can do, depending on your interest.

Levels of
Volunteer Advocate Skills

Rookie
Make first contact with elected official.
Deliver organization's message.
Understand need for accuracy.
Respond to action alerts.
Believe lobbying is honorable, effective.
Become personally effective.
Get to know staff.
Write letter to editor.

Pro
Build personal, supportive relationship.
Call, contact, write, fax systematically.
Become trusted information source to politicians.
Report to HQ and discuss results.
Participate in campaigns.
Recruit others to lobby.
Politician knows your name, organization, issues.
Give personal money.
Submit Op-ed piece.

Hall of Famer
Become trusted advisor to elected official.
Politician and staff call you and request information.
Testify at hearings; talk with media.
Gather intelligence and spot trends.
Raise money for PAC.
Organize home-based fundraisers.
Find allies for coalition.
Meet with editorial board.

Getting Craft your Message to Penetrate the Clutter

What will make your message stand out?

In Washington DC and your state, politicians have no back burner. They only deal with things that are hot, burning and immediate. Back when President Bush was trying to do something about Social Security, a member of his own party, Rep. Rob Simmons (CT), had this to say: "Why stir up a political hornet's nest…when there is no urgency? When does the program go belly up? 2042. I will be dead by then." (The Washington Post, Jan 11, 2005)

There are two kinds of messages to get through to your elected official. I call these the "macro message" and the "micro message." The macro message is important to the state (or nation) and is delivered best by the professional lobbyist or leaders of your state or national organization. The micro message is important to you and me and to the people in your district.

Micro Message

Your part, as the volunteer advocate, is to help develop and deliver the micro message to your elected official. In most cases, it works best if the volunteer lobbyist deals only with the micro message. You are letting your elected official know your issue is important to people in the district. This way you are dealing with things you know well.

Indeed, you are an expert; you know things the professional lobbyist doesn't. This approach also means you don't have to know the technicalities of legislation or the legislative process (although that can be useful).

First we'll look at how to construct a message, then how to deliver it.

I've surveyed hundreds of state and federal officeholders asking them this question: "What do you want from volunteer

I've surveyed hundreds of state and federal officeholders asking them this question: "What do you want from volunteer lobbyists?" The answers come back clear and consistent: "Be accurate, be brief and tell me something new."

Be Accurate

Accuracy means you never go beyond what you know to be absolutely, mathematically true. If you ever exaggerate, distort, misstate facts or the other side's position, you are dead. Neither the elected official nor his staff will ever listen to you again.

Professional lobbyists know this rule and obey it. Volunteers sometimes don't understand it and get carried away in their enthusiasm. While they don't actually lie, they may not present the whole picture or they may exaggerate. It's easy when you care a lot, but it's fatal.

Fortunately there's an easy way out. Do not go beyond what you know to be absolutely true. Then, if you're doing a good job, you will get a great opportunity – you will be asked a question you cannot answer. And what do you say? "I don't know...but I will find out" or even better, "May I have our professional lobbyist call you?"

The second answer works better because it sets up a warm call between your professional lobbyist and the elected official. You complete an important triangle consisting of the elected official, yourself (the constituent) and the professional. Generally speaking, it's better to leave complicated technical details to the professionals. That's their job; they are likely to have a better grasp of it and they will deliver a consistent message.

Your job is to deliver your part of the message: how the issue affects you, your practice and the people in your community. You want your elected officials to know that you have a headache and what it will take to cure it. You want them to know that your issue, your problem, is important to their voters.

If they don't believe the people who put them in office care about the issue, they are free to ignore the professional lobbyist. So knowing that people in the district have a headache is the first step to getting relief.

Indeed, your own legislator may never need or want to know the details because your solution, your bill or whatever will be handled in a committee of which he is not a member. But he can be powerful on your behalf conveying his interest to the action committee and leadership.

Your professional lobbyist can present both the larger picture as it relates to public policy and politics and the smaller picture of technical details. Your professional is like a coach, setting game strategy and calling plays from the sideline, but only you and other grassroots activists can carry the ball and score, because only you can make it important to elected officials.

Be Brief

Learn to take no longer than thirty seconds to state what you want and why you want it. If you force yourself to deliver your message in thirty seconds, you will boil it down to its essence. If you can't get their attention in thirty seconds, you probably haven't focused your message.

Often you don't get more than thirty seconds. Politicians are busy and always have a line of people waiting to talk with them. You may run into them at the chamber of commerce or at a party. I've seen more than one very effective communication as a volunteer walked from the elevator to the office with an elected official.

To develop a winning thirty-second message, ask yourself two questions:
1. What do I want?
2. What key reason can I cite to win support?

You want your elected official to support your position. Sometimes you will have a specific bill number. Even when you do, make sure he understands the concepts or fundamental ideas you support because specific bills can change, disappear and merge.

Start with a focused opening that hooks the politician – what you want and why you want it. Use the format: We want _____ because _____.

Imagine you are a group of physicians, for example. You could say, "We want Medicaid reimbursement increased at least to the breakeven point so we can treat people without losing money even though we won't make any."

Although it is helpful to give a complete briefing on all aspects of your issue, that isn't usually necessary. Your main goal is to wake up your elected official and let him know that this matters to people in the district. Give him a sense of what you want, why you want it, who it affects and how.

Then, if he is still listening, you move to the hardest part of the message.

Tell Me Something New

Unless your representative has just been elected, chances are good that he's heard it all before. There are very few new issues. Anyone who has been in office for a complete election cycles will glaze over the moment your mouth opens unless you can say something he hasn't heard before.

You will have to work hard to get him to listen.

In the case of a newly elected person, the challenge is to educate him from ground zero. Most likely he will be eager to hear you out. In either case, the greater challenge is to cause him to remember and care. You see, the day after the election, they all come down with a disease called TIO: terminal information overload.

They are swamped with issue papers, letters and personal appeals from everybody with a cause. They get on every mailing list, and at first they try to absorb as much information as possible.

They quickly learn – the smart ones at least – that they have to choose very carefully and focus their efforts in order to get anything done. They can't give equal attention to everyone and they can't even give attention to all good causes. They have to pick causes that are important to them and to those who got them elected.

Your job, as a volunteer, is to cut through the clutter with something your official will remember and recognize as important. The antidote for terminal information overload is the anecdote – a story about a living, breathing (or, if it fits, dead) person affected by the issue. It needs to have as much detail as possible to make it credible: names, dates, addresses, ages, occupations – anything that will make the person real.

Here's a great example of a specific powerful story that was in the news in Austin TX: Just nine people accounted for nearly 2,700 of the emergency room visits in the Austin area during the past six years at a cost of $3 million to taxpayers and others, according to a report. The patients went to hospital emergency rooms 2,678 times from 2003 through 2008, said the report from the nonprofit Integrated Care Collaboration, a group of health care providers who care for low-income and uninsured patients.

Watch What You Say

In the example of Medicaid reimbursement you have to get to what I call the dollars and cents of healthcare. Share a true personal experience from your own life and practice. In addition to bringing the issue to life and putting a face on it, the anecdotes serve another purpose: proving the problem exists. That's important.

One of my clients told me about a group of people in Colorado who were trying to get legislation passed to prevent "takings." People in the "takings movement," as it is called, believe the government should not take property or reduce the value of property without fair compensation.

A group in Colorado had introduced its legislation and had even gone so far as to get a hearing. They made their presentation and the first question they were asked was, "Can you give us an example that happened in Colorado of a taking such as you oppose?"

The spokesmen looked around, paused, scratched their heads – no, they couldn't. They were laughed out of the room. The kind of thing they opposed doesn't happen in Colorado. I'm told that to this day the lobbyists at the capitol jokingly call out to the lobbyist from the takings group, "Hey Bob, got your anecdote yet?"

(For several years I told this story in my seminars across the country, based on the story from a client who said he was there. Not long ago, unbeknownst to me, the lobbyist in the story was in my audience. Later he came up and confirmed that it happened just as I had been told, much to his embarrassment. As for his real name, my lips are sealed.)

The real-life stories and anecdotes that illuminate your issue are important for several reasons. If you can't come up with real-life situations, it may look as though you have no problem. The stories dramatize your issue, make it memorable, give it credibility and cut through the information overload. You take the statistical abstract and turn it into real people.

They Like Pressing The Flesh

Politicians are people-people. While they are interested in numbers and the broad scope and sweep of things, they respond more to living, breathing people in their district who vote and who they can help. That's why the volunteer's job – your job – is to humanize the issue.

You need to provide the illuminating anecdote that personalizes the issue. You need to tell the memorable story that will stimulate emotion and action. This is something professional lobbyists often cannot come up with because they don't live with the problem.

For example, banks have fought long and hard for the right to sell insurance. As I worked with a group of bankers to find that illuminating anecdote, most were talking vaguely about helping their customers, having a level playing field or offering competition to the insurance companies.

All this was good, but it was abstract and the same old argument. We couldn't find a way to make it come to life.

Then a woman told this story:

"Our bank is in a poor neighborhood. Two times in the last year we have held the accounts for fund-raising drives to pay for funerals for teenagers who were killed. This is a minority neighborhood and funerals are really important. The families had no money to pay for a funeral. Insurance agents don't come to this neighborhood. Since we are already in the neighborhood and have relationships, it would really help these people if we could offer them burial insurance policies."

Now that is a compelling story. If I were campaigning to pass a bill to let banks sell insurance, I would put this woman and her story into a video and also make sure she tells it to politicians.

Do You Have Any Real People

I've already mentioned Ralph Wright, former Speaker of the Vermont House of Representatives. In his book "All Politics Is Personal" he tells the story of one representative he worked with:

"Most of the time he drove me crazy with his 'no-tax, no-spend' votes, but I learned over time I could get him to vote for something if I could place the problem right smack in front of him. I don't mean the issue, rather, the person who would feel the impact of a vote. If I wanted his help on a foster program, for example, I would arrange for him to coincidentally run into a foster kid whom I just happened to have with me. People touched his heart, not theories. Corc [the representative] could be trusted, not if WE believed in the deal, but only if HE believed in it."

When you put real people into a story, you make the case for your issue. You tell them something new. The issue of giving banks the right to sell insurance has been around for many years. There isn't anything new you can say about it and there's probably nothing new to say about Medicaid or Medicare.

But you can offer a new story that illuminates the issue in a new way. You can win sympathy and you can get your elected official to remember and care.

Make your story as specific as possible. Use real names, dates and situations. If you've done a good job, the politician may want your help getting in touch with the people involved. Do it.

Remember, to make your micro message successful, (1) be accurate, (2) be brief, and (3) tell him something new.

Macro Message

This is the message you must convey to enough people in the legislature or Congress to get that critical 50% plus one. Usually this will be the result of a thorough deliberative process involving lots of people, lots of fact gathering and a careful assessment of what is desirable and what is possible.

Your association will develop a consensus as to what the macro message is. Sometimes I call this the "case statement." It spells out the fundamental reasons why politicians should support your cause.

A winning macro message starts with a firm moral, practical, and political foundation. Without all three parts of this foundation, it's tough to win. The stronger you can make each part, the more likely you are to get what you want. You must demonstrate clearly that your cause is moral, practical and political – or at least make it look as moral, practical and political as possible.

Three Successful Elements

You and I both know there are lots of laws and regulations passed that would fail these tests. Conversely, many ideas people would like to pass into law seem to be good ideas, but they never get anywhere. Much depends on how you "frame" the issue – taking what you have and making it look like what everybody wants. You do it deliberately, step-by-step, looking for those three elements.

1. Moral

Is it right? Is it a good thing to do? Is it in the public interest? Can you show that it is? You have to make the case. Take, for example, smoking and the regulation of cigarettes.

If you are a cigarette company, you do not argue that cigarettes are good for people. Nobody would buy that. You can't win arguing the health issue.

And simply saying "it's legal" isn't much help either, because the response will be, "Okay, let's make it illegal." So how can you frame the issue to win?

What do the tobacco companies argue? You've seen the ads. It's not about health; it's about individual rights. You have a right to smoke. You have the right to choose.

This is called "framing the issue" and you see it all the time on television. Usually someone will say something like, "I'm glad you asked that, Dan, because that's not the issue. The real issue is..."

Once you frame the issue correctly, it is easier for a politician to support you. Your elected representative cannot argue that cigarettes are healthy. But he can take your side and argue that people have a right to choose.

You and your professional lobbyists must frame the issue in such a way that the politician can take your side and still occupy the moral high ground. The politician needs you to give him that logical framework, that position he can stand on when he answers questions from opponents, family and the media. You must provide the answer that allows the politician to take your side and be proud and public about it.

2. Practical

Will it work? If you want to eliminate a regulation or create one, and if you have shown me that it is the right thing to do, you still have to demonstrate to me that it will do the job and be cost-effective.

For example, many of my nursing home clients battle with the government every budget cycle to get more money for the Medicaid program.

The challenge is to show that it is necessary to put more money in to maintain adequate care for poor people. It's tough because you come very close to saying that if you don't get more money, the quality of care in nursing homes will fall below standards, which no one wants to say.

One strategy we used in Florida was to show – using the government's own numbers – that about half the nursing homes were operating at a loss.

We argued that there was no way they could stay in business while operating at a loss and, unless the state wanted to set up its own tax payer supported nursing home system, something had to give.

Make Your Story Come To Life

It worked for several reasons. We had credible numbers because the nursing home cost reports are all audited. We could also argue that the alternative would be to set up government nursing homes, which most people believe will be less efficient than those run by private enterprise.

Practicality is important for any issue. If you want to reduce the paperwork involved in making loans, you have to show that the consumer will still be fully informed about interest rates and the real cost of the loan.

Got problem with Medicare or Medicaid reimbursement? Show me the effect of current law or regulations, what a change would do and how it will work.

I once had a wonderful testimonial from an orthopedic surgeon who, because of liability issues, had to stop operating on spines. He said there was no surgeon for 200 miles who could do these procedures and the wait time was about one year. That's a good demonstration of lack of access.

But you must help with that part. It's not your elected official's job to come up with the rationale for what you want.

3. Political

Does what you want have or potentially have widespread support? Who cares and how much? Politicians often measure that by how many people they are hearing from and who those people are. Their own voters? People they know? Supporters?

Did your allies send an e-mail or call? Did they show up in person at a town hall meeting? Did they write once or many times? How much you care will be measured in part by the effort you make delivering your message. Were you willing to travel to the Capitol?

If so, that makes a statement about your concern and commitment.

Your politician will wonder, "Who else is with you? What organizations?"

As a matter of practical reality, elected officials are only going to put their energy and reputation behind issues that have some chance of winning.

They are not in the habit of supporting losing causes, no matter how correct. You must show that they can get the 50% plus one they will need every step of the way and how they are going to get it. So much for the message. Just frame your issue so it looks moral, practical and political.

Be accurate. Be brief. Tell them something new. Then deliver the message.

What Works And What Doesn't

In our surveys of elected officials, we have asked what are the most effective methods to communicate. Generally they say they would like to have more good communications from constituents, and they have strong feelings about what works best.

What I say below may conflict with what you are hearing from some organization asking you to take action. It's true that anything you do has some impact, just as the flapping of a butterfly wing in China may affect weather in your town.

My suggestion is that you focus on things that we know work and work well. First, let's look at some things that don't work particularly well.

Petitions Pa-Toohey

A guy came to my office the other day with a petition. The petition was on its way to Congress. The petition urged members of Congress to allow small business people to fully deduct the cost of health insurance. I think that makes sense and I was happy to sign. I also noticed that this guy worked for an association of small businesses and he now had my address and phone number. Sure enough, he tried to get me to join.

I have no quarrel with what he was doing, although I suspect he was as motivated by a desire to sign up members as he was to fight for the rights of small business. That's because if he had been serious about the issue, he would not have used a petition.

Petitions just don't work as a way to influence legislators. I have asked hundreds of politicians and they all confirm: petitions are next to worthless as an influencing tactic.

Suppose you have 5,000 names on a petition. I'm your senator and you give it to me and say, "Here are 5,000 people who support the idea that small business owners ought to be able to fully deduct the cost of health insurance." I take the petition in my hand. I say thank you.

Then what? What am I supposed to do? Who are these people? Do they vote? Do they live in my district? Are they real? Did they have any clue what they were signing?

I can tell you what your elected official and his staff will say. They think people will sign a petition without reading it. They think that even if the petitioner read it and understood it, merely signing a list does not represent a serious commitment. This is especially true of mass campaigns that sign up people in shopping centers. Therefore, politicians pay little or no attention to a petition. A petition with 5,000 names is worth no more than one letter, often less.

If petitions don't work, why do organizations carry on petition campaigns? They do it to enlist, motivate, activate and energize the people who sign – to get publicity and visibility. Petitions have significant value in recruiting activists, getting public recognition and other things, but in the battle to influence politicians directly, they are virtually worthless.

Remember, politicians suffer from a disease called terminal information overload. They are overwhelmed with input from all kinds of people, and most of it is impersonal and not very thoughtful. It's difficult to imagine anything more impersonal and thoughtless than a petition.

Mass Mail, E-mail And Telemarketing

In Washington DC and in your state capitol, the political pros distinguish between real communication and fake communication by using the terms "grassroots" and "astro turf."

Astro turf is the derogatory term for the mass-generated, impersonal faxes, form letters, e-mails and phone calls stimulated by corporations, associations and their PR firms. An example of this is when some associations hire telemarketing firms in Washington to call their members, give them a quick briefing, then hook them up with a member of Congress.

This can backfire in a big way. When the person in the district talks with a staff member, it only takes a couple of questions to find out that the caller is on the phone because some hired agency in Washington called. The caller really doesn't know much about the issue. It's embarrassing to the caller and to the staff member. Staff reacts negatively because they have wasted their time.

Fake Is Fake And Soon Outed

In one infamous case from August 2009, Bonner & Associates, one of the Washington PR companies who regularly gin up grass roots, was busted for sending fake letters from community groups to a member of Congress. The company blamed and fired a low-level temp for sending the letters. Their client, American Coalition for Clean Coal Electricity, though apparently innocent, suffered a major black eye.

The perception is growing among members of Congress and staff that this sort of thing goes on regularly, making them more and more skeptical of any communications they get from people they don't know.

The same thing is true with computer-generated faxes, e-mails and letters. The staff who receive them quickly detect that the message is from a computer, not a person. They not only discount it but get annoyed because they have to deal with what is essentially meaningless communication.

In a variation on this theme, some associations set up e-mail communications and telephones at their conventions. They rope in people and tell them who to write and what to write. The phone calls, faxes and e-mails pour into Washington.

In Washington they say, "Oh, yeah, more mail from the convention." They answer it, usually, but what effect do you think it has? It's similar to what one politician described. He said he could always tell when a preacher has stirred his flock because on Wednesday he will get a load of mail. Although he answers it politely, he doesn't think there's much commitment there and it doesn't sway him.

Raising Money vs. Political Impact

I put myself on the lists for many political organizations just to see what they are doing. I frequently get e-mails asking me to e-mail my members of Congress and, oh by the way, please contribute.

It's a good way to raise money, I guess, since they keep doing it, but the political impact is close to zero. If these techniques don't work, why do people use them? Several realities drive this sometimes counterproductive activity: Organizations need to show their stakeholders they are doing something and it's an easy way to get people involved. The preachers need to stir up their flock and help them feel they are doing something. It's easy.

The companies providing these services do a good job of selling and professional lobbyists are all looking for an easy way to get influence. The folks involved are fooled into believing they have had significant input and can take smug satisfaction that they have told off the politicians. (This may lead to frustration when it doesn't work.)

There are instances in which an overwhelming number of people participate and the pressure is too intense to resist, even though the commitment is shallow. In one famous case, Congress wanted to take quarterly tax deductions from savings accounts. The banks got millions of customers to send in preprinted cards. It worked.

All the people ranting against changes in health care insurance had some impact. But when the dust settles, the people who show up with relationships and specific, workable ideas will ultimately prevail.

Action, Re-Action – Anything Might Work, Once

More recently, Congress at first balked at the financial bail-out bill because of a tsunami coming in from irate radio talk show listeners.

If you shoot enough BBs at a brick wall, you can eventually break it down. But it takes a lot of BBs. Only a few issues and a few organizations are capable of stimulating that kind of response, and they can't do it often.

Interestingly, right after the talk show ditto-heads swamped Congress in opposition to the bail-out bill, the chambers of commerce and small business and other communities counter-reacted and prevailed because they are connected to the political system and they used more personal techniques.

It's true that everything and anything you do has some impact. It is also true that you can, with enough effort and the right techniques, stir up meaningful communication. If you can cause constituents to have thoughtful, personal communication with the person they vote for, it will work.

But most massive efforts produce only shallow, hit or miss letters and phone calls with little result. All I can say is, every member of Congress or state legislature and every staff person I have talked with, hundreds of them, say these mass techniques have little or no positive effect, and they often have a negative effect. I believe in using techniques that we know will have a strong impact.

Messages – What Do They Want

So what do elected officials and their staffs want? Thoughtful, personal communications from people who can help them get re-elected. Something that shows a real person in the district cares. They want to know who cares and how much. Show you care about them, you care about your issue and you care a lot.

Letters (or e-mail if you already have a relationship)

Politicians tell me (and numerous scientific surveys show) that thoughtful, personal contact within a relationship, however you make it, is the most powerful contact. After face-to-face, I give the edge to postal letters, especially at the state level. As for Congress, because of the ricin poison and anthrax scares, postal mail can take forever to arrive. When it does get there, one chief of staff told me, it is often "fried," that is, brittle, because it has been treated to kill anything in it.

Unless you hand-carry your mail, it's problematic. In the near future I expect that everything sent will be scanned into electronic form and forwarded to Congress, so postal mail has significant limitations. That makes e-mail and faxes your best options.

You can also hand carry a letter to the local office of your member of Congress and it will be sent in the regular packet, which goes to Washington perhaps once a week

But you have to be careful and persistent if your e-mail is to even get through. Generally, before you can send an e-mail to a member of the House, you go to their Web site and fill in a long form that includes your name, address, city, e-mail address and phone number. They tend to ask for your ZIP code first and reject you if you don't give one in the district. To weed out the liars, they respond with a letter to whatever address you sent in. They almost all state up front they only can deal with communications from their own voters.

I have found that sending messages this way is useless. I get nothing but rote responses, if that, from my own member of Congress, Alan Boyd. I consider him to be a hardworking, effective member of Congress. I have shaken his hand and contributed to his campaign.

In May of 2009 I got this email from his office:

Dear Mr. Blackwell:

Thank you for contacting me. My office had some issues with our mailing system earlier in the year which has resulted in a delay of a handful of letters and unfortunately, yours is one of them.

Should you still have concerns that you expressed, please do not hesitate to contact my Legislative Director, Kara Stencel, in my Washington, DC office.

I apologize for the delay and please continue to write to me, and I encourage you to sign up for my e-newsletter by visiting my website at www.house.gov/boyd

Sincerely, F. Allen Boyd, Jr.
Member of Congress

AB:ks
Confirmation# 1280231

Notice this did not mention the topic of my letter.

This lame statement "My office had some issues..." makes me wonder. They knew I had sent something, but they didn't know what it was? How could this be? How many communications did they lose? Is it credible that they lost only a "handful"?

According to one study, electronic messages to the House doubled to 99 million from 2000 to 2004. In the Senate, the number of e-mails more than tripled to 83 million, and it's growing geometrically.

Grassroots Activist Code Of Practice

A study by the Congress Online Project was funded by a grant from the Pew Charitable Trusts and conducted by George Washington University and the Congressional Management Foundation. Here is what they recommended:

First, grassroots activists should adopt a code of conduct to engage in electronic lobbying practices that:

- Targets individuals' own Members of Congress and only their own Members of Congress

- Sends meaningful messages, not "electronic postcards"

- Avoids sending duplicate messages from the same person

- Encourages people to speak in their own words

- Does not foster the expectation that citizens should correspond with – and expect a response from – any Member of Congress with whom they choose to communicate

- Provides complete identification information, including name, address, zip code, and e-mail address.

Second, citizens must recognize that congressional offices are not, and cannot be, capable of responding electronically to every American and limit their e-mails to communicating with only their elected representatives. Due to the large and growing volumes of e-mail congressional offices are receiving, electronic communication should be confined to Member-constituent communications.

Third, both the House and Senate should consider increasing the budgets of Hill offices to help them manage the demands of e-mail, or develop other means of providing these offices with the assistance they need to solve this problem.

Fourth, congressional offices must expedite the transition to operating efficient and responsive e-mail systems. The dated practices offices are adhering to become less practical with each passing month, as greater numbers of Americans become "wired." Continuing to process incoming e-mail manually is a costly drain on office time and resources. Continuing to answer e-mail with paper fails to meet the timeliness and responsiveness constituents expect. Continuing to cling to misconceptions about e-mail causes congressional offices to appear behind the times and resistant to change.

In this congressional e-mail standoff, there are no winners, only losers. The interests of no party – congressional offices, constituents, the general public, and public interest groups – are being met. Electronic communication has the potential to strengthen our democracy. It holds the promise of creating greater openness and a broader dialogue between Members of Congress and their constituents. To realize this potential, however, the public, activists, and Members of Congress must all become better users of the powerful tools they possess.

I believe the evidence shows the only way e-mail works is when you send it to a person you know, confirm they got it and make sure you get a meaningful response.

Others conclude the same thing. An article in The Washington Post by John Schwartz was headlined, "Sometimes E-mail Just Doesn't Deliver."

Schwartz quoted activist Jonah Seiger, who works for a consulting firm called Mindshare Internet Campaigns: To make an impression in a legislator's office, Seiger said, "it is very important to make noise. E-mail doesn't do that."

Electronic mail, Seiger said, "has no weight. It has no mass. It comes in quietly and gets filtered by computers."

American University and Bonner Associates did a study on e-mail and found that it is substantially discounted. One flaw that staff people cite about e-mail is that e-mail addresses don't tell where a person lives. A majority of staffers I talk to disregard e-mail. They delete it or send a bland automatic response, unless they have some clear indication the person lives in the district.

Almost every member of Congress has a web site and on that web site they stress that you should not correspond unless you are a constituent.

One politician recently told me he never responds to e-mail. "If I do, they send me another note. I respond again. They respond again. It never ends. So I just send a letter and that's it. That's all I have time for."

But this is changing rapidly and e-mail is clearly the wave of the future. It just works too well. When you are using e-mail and have the address of a person in Washington (not the form you fill in on their site), it is even more important to signal in the subject line that you live in the district – something like "Message From Joel Blackwell in Arlington." Give your name, town and address right up front of the message so they can see it.

However, the politicians, especially in Washington, prefer you to go through their website and use their form.

I must say, however, I have had very poor results using these forms, often getting no response at all or just an automatic response. I think the volume means they often just disappear.

Sending a message from your association's website is useful, because this allows the association to track it. But again these systems produce very weak, impersonal input. However you communicate, make sure the association gets a copy of your message and the response.

That said, I'm not a fan of e-mail and it certainly has its limitations. Capital Advantage, one of the pioneers of email systems for companies and associations to communicate to Congress, said in July 2009 19 million emails had already been sent that year.

In January the company posted the latest summary year as 2007 and listed this many messages of all kinds to Congress through Capital Advantage:

Over 14.5 million constituent messages.
E-mail: over 13.5 million
Fax: over 220,000
Printed: over 625,000
Hand-Delivered: over 400,000

Note the comparatively small number of faxes and hand delivered letters. Which pile would you rather be in?

There is a more subtle downside to your e-mail to Congress, and that's the mob it arrives with. You can go to Congress.org and see what people are sending to Congress. Here is part of one sample I picked at random, unchanged from the original:

...There is an organized evil it has always been here and is approaching critical mass. who, why, how, where, when —I don't know, and i don't care, someday we may know, the point is, its here and we have to stop it. After WWII this evil concentrated in two places America and Israel. Jews were chosen to actualize this evil, the covenant that they made

was with this evil and not god. The god depicted in the bible, is this evil, the whole judo-christian religion is descendant of this evil...

The editor in me cringed, but I put it to you as it was sent. This particular screed went on for more than 3500 words. It is unfortunately typical of a lot of the messages pouring into Washington and your state capitol. Clearly some people are using Congress for group therapy. I worry that your e-mail, coming between two of these, may be somewhat diminished.

However, if you have a relationship and are known to the person you are e-mailing and if you confirm they received it, e-mail can work. If it's working for you, fine, use it. If not, try something else.

Historically, it's surprising how many politicians use very similar words when they answer the question, "What is the most powerful communication, the one you are most likely to respond to?" Their reply is usually, "A letter written on ruled paper in pencil by a little old lady."

I don't suggest you do that because it might come across as phony. (On the other hand, it would stand out. For example, handwritten thank-you notes have enormous penetrating power.) But the old-lady letter symbolizes what they are looking for: a real person with a real problem who cares a lot and lives in the district.

Do You Show A Serious Commitment?

A person who sits down to write a letter is expressing a serious commitment. It takes longer to write a letter than make a phone call. Few people send a thoughtful, personal letter, so they stand out when they arrive.

For years I have given the same advice: Make your letter one page, one issue. Just tell the politicians what you want and why you want it. However, as I continue probing to find what works best, I get more examples convincing me that a thoughtful, personal, really good long letter will get really good, long consideration. Staff and elected officials alike have cited examples of single letters that were so compelling they had to hold a meeting to answer them. The letter raised good issues and made them think.

A long, thoughtful letter carries a heavy weight of commitment that must be answered. It also stands out because almost all others are short. But it must be a good letter, full of facts and persuasive argument and meaningful detail from the politician's district or state.

Some kinds of letters don't work, however. If you get an action alert from your association, personalize it into your own words on your own letterhead, using your own examples. Many groups nowadays send out talking points and ask you to select your own and rewrite them.

That's a good idea.

Some people take an action alert or sample form letter, write their legislator's name at the top and put their name at the bottom and send it.

Don't laugh. I have seen letters that arrived in Washington with a computer code salutation (Name) (Address) (City) (State) (Zip) crossed out and the recipient's name written in. At the bottom, still shining through the ink, were the words (Your Signature), dutifully crossed out with a real signature nearby. Needless to say, that doesn't meet the standard for thoughtful, personal communication.

Know What Works For Sure And Do That First

Some people used to use preprinted postcards that way, but hardly anyone does anymore. You just sign your name and drop it in the mailbox. I'm not saying it has no effect. Enough postcards at least indicate that the issue has a constituency willing to sign a postcard. It may get some attention. But it only works if you can produce tens of thousands of those, and most of us aren't usually engaged in a mass campaign that can produce those kinds of numbers.

- What works is a personal, thoughtful communication from a constituent.

- Your letter can be as simple as three paragraphs:

- Tell your politician what you want,

- Cite an example from the district,

- Say you'll check back in two weeks.

Will you get a form letter back? Probably. That's okay, particularly if it seems supportive. If you get a letter back that is so vague it gives you no clue, here's a secret: Send another letter, only this time, in the last paragraph, ask a question he cannot answer in a form letter. Keep it up until you get an answer. It may take a while and a phone call. Sometimes a politician is trying not to state a position or give you an answer.

More likely an overwhelmed junior staff member glanced at your letter to get the subject and hit the print button on a canned response.

A good communication, at the very least, may make some staff person think through and perhaps have a discussion with a more senior person. Getting them to construct the form letter is a good first step toward winning support. The presence of a specific form letter is a sure sign they are hearing from the district. (Their form letter to you is good. Your form letter to them is bad.)

Give Key Locator Information Up Front

Here's another secret for a powerful letter and especially an e-mail. Begin your letter by accurately stating the number of the district you live in. (You live in a numbered district for your state senator and representative and federal House of Representatives.

For United States senators, indicate your state by your address.) When you do this, you automatically lift yourself out of the pack of passionate but uninformed constituents.

You show you are politically savvy and a serious player. Not one voter in 10,000 knows the number of the district they live in, even among those who know the name of their representative (and that's a very small group too). Believe me, those elected officials know their district number and will respect you when you speak their language.

Another tip: When you send your letter, make sure to give them permission and a phone number to call you late at night or on the weekend, and include your number at home, particularly if your politician is in session.

Elected officials work long days; often the only time they have to call is on weekends and at night. Your willingness to do this not only makes their lives easier, but it also shows that you are committed beyond normal working hours. If you have a private number or cell phone number, give it to them and tell them that's what it is.

Netroots And The Influence Of Bloggers

The Internet has definitely changed campaigns as shown by Barrack Obama's win.

The role of bloggers in producing news, debunking rumors, spreading rumors and raising money has been much commented on. You can get a full review of the phenomenon in the book, "Bloggers On The Bus," by Boehlert.

The question I have is how will Facebook, MySpace, Flickr, Twitter and YouTube impact the legislative process. My guess is, not much at all for 99% percent of the issues that affect the delivery of health care.

All these techniques begin very quickly to look to elected officials like pre-printed post cards coming through the Internet by the thousands.

There are too many to read, from too many people outside the district and, often, too crazy, hysterical, shrill and threatening.

But smart people may yet find a way.

The blog Firedoglake by Jane Hamsher posted this announcement in July 2009:

> Max Bernstein and James Boyce of dotPAC are running a campaign of Facebook ads in the districts of the 7 Blue Dog obstructionists , asking people who are constituents to call or leave messages on their Facebook walls. I asked the dotPAC folks how much it would cost to run these ads effectively, and they said $35 per day per representative. As someone who looks constantly for effective ways to build pressure within the districts of people who can be awfully hard to target, this is really smart, microtargeted and cost-effective effort. People around here know that I don't jump on campaigns lightly -- most of the traditional ways that liberals do advocacy are in need of serious re-examination because they just plain don't work. But I gave $100 myself to this one. I think it's a great idea and recommend it highly.

The seven were Mike Ross, John Barrow, Baron Hill, Bart Gordon, Jim Matheson, Charlie Melancon Jr. and Zack Space.

She included a link to the dotPAC donation page. About a day later the site listed donations of about $8,000, enough to run quite a few ads.

I checked Mike Ross's site and there were about 40 comments, mostly supportive, so it's hard to say what effect, if any the ads were having.

Will Your Message Be Diss'd Even If Noticed?

Even if you assume lots of people in his district responded and identified themselves as constituents and were believed, the number is not likely to be great enough to sway him and will likely be cancelled out by people on the other side.

I like the idea of targeting ads to stimulate constituents to contact elected officials, but my guess is that emails from unknowns of unknown origin will likely be dismissed.

In August of 2009 groups of spirited activists set out to, shall we say, enliven town hall meetings during the August recess. Some were exposed as paid outside agitators, but many came out of a genuine passion for some cause.

You can criticize their tactics and their lack of courtesy, but they showed up and probably had some impact, although it's hard to know what they were for or against based on their signs and shouted slogans.

Many were energized through the Internet and used texting and Tweeting to communicate. But did they change the mind of any member of Congress? I didn't see any indication they did by those boisterous, intrusive tactics. Bullying seldom works and I don't recommend it.

Will Obama's Mighty Wind Blow?

On the other side, there is Barack Obama's much vaunted grassroots operation which played a huge role in getting him elected. His organization had millions of people responding to e-mailed action alerts with action on the ground.

But things were different when it came to the healthcare debate, as shown in this report from the New York Times:

"Mr. Obama engendered such passion last year that his allies believed they were on the verge of creating a movement that could be mobilized again. But if a week's worth of events are any measure here in Iowa, it may not be so easy to reignite the machine that overwhelmed Republicans a year ago.

"More than a dozen campaign volunteers, precinct captains and team leaders from all corners of Iowa, who dedicated a large share of their time in 2007 and 2008 to Mr. Obama, said in interviews this week that they supported the president completely but were taking a break from politics and were not active members of Organizing for America." (Aug. 15, 2009)

Faxes

I've become a big fan of faxes. They are fast and easy. The only drawbacks are the quality depends on the printer where they arrive and they will be in black and white, whereas your letterhead, particularly if you are writing on company letterhead, may have more impact because it is in color.

Elected officials tell me they like faxes because they are easy to work with. They often just write a note on them and fax them back. One thing that seems to work well is to send something timely from the newspaper with a note on it. Chances are good you will get there before the papers do and your note takes on added value. You are helping them and they will remember you.

When you send a fax, send to the right person by name. This means finding out who on staff handles your issues. Then call to make sure the right person got it. Congressional offices are not always the most organized places and paperwork gets mislaid a lot. Sometimes faxes don't arrive because of technical problems and sometimes they just get lost. The person you are sending to may be gone. Your follow-up call gives two impressions and doubles the chance that the right person will see it.

Almost every computer today has the ability to send a fax straight out of your word processing software such as Microsoft Word.

You must be hooked up to a phone line, but you can do this easily by unplugging the line to your phone and plugging it in to your computer. Then you simply hit the print button and choose fax as the printer. This also allows you to easily create a personal letterhead if you don't want to use your office letterhead in a political letter. Because it comes straight out of your computer, it gives the best possible quality coming out of the fax.

When I send letters like this, I sign my name using a script font in 24-point type. It looks like this:

Joel Blackwell

That may not matter, but to me, it looks more personal than a typed name.

Phone

Legislators love the phone because they can have a quick two-way dialogue, if you can get past the staff.

But it's often hard to get them during office hours. If you call, it helps to make notes about what you want to say before you call. Here's a checklist for your lobbying phone call.

1. Primary objective: What do I want to happen?

2. Secondary objective: What will I settle for?

3. What points am I going to make to get the results I want?

4. What open-ended questions will I ask to keep the conversation going?

5. What exact words will I use (write them down) to ask for what I want?

6. What is the likely response when I close by asking for what I want, and how do I respond?

7. What questions will I be asked?

One thing I observe when I watch people make phone calls is that they often get nervous and talk too fast. You don't have the advantage of using your own body language or reading theirs, so slow down. Speak distinctly.

Make sure they know who you are not only by giving your name slowly and clearly, but also by anchoring them with an image they will remember: "We talked at the chamber meeting in April" or "I sent the article on taxes two weeks ago." They get so many calls that if they don't know you like a family member they may not understand who you are.

If you make your pitch and he isn't asking questions, get off the line – you haven't engaged him. Follow up with an e-mail or fax. Reiterate what you meant to say and what you thought you heard in response.

Many times you will get voice mail and need to leave a message. I love voice mail because I've got my message ready and can be pretty sure I have their attention for thirty seconds until I leave the number.

I state my name and phone number v-e-r-y slowly at the end of my message and then repeat it. It is amazing how many people compliment me on this. In contrast, I have gotten many voice mails where the caller, so used to leaving his own number, speeds up and leaves something I can barely understand. So make sure you give your name and number carefully and slowly. Repeat the number, especially if you are on a cell phone. You want your politician to call back.

Preparing For Person-To-Person Communication

While I am a great believer in letters (properly delivered), nothing beats an eyeball-to-eyeball conversation. Politicians often tell me, "It's hard to say no when you're looking them in the eye."

Before you have an oral communication – in person or by phone – I recommend you take out a 4 x 6 card. Write down specifically what you want to happen. For example: "I want you to vote for House Bill x."

Then give three good reasons why your elected representative should support it – three ways it will make a difference in the district. Write down an example of how it's working, or not working, or will work. This example should be concrete, specific and about a specific person you can name (the anecdote).

For example, I was working with convenience store operators who wanted to pass a state law requiring mandatory ID checks for the age of any person buying tobacco products. There was a law in place making it illegal to sell tobacco products to anyone under eighteen, but it was often ignored.

The police had just run a sting operation in which they dressed up a mature looking sixteen-year-old girl and sent her around to buy cigarettes, which she did. Then they arrested the clerks.

I felt the store owners could make a good case that it was unrealistic to ask minimum wage clerks to be the enforcers and to make the decision who to ask. It was especially unfair to punish them for what could be an honest mistake. It would be much easier to make everyone show an ID.

Your Focus Determines Their Interest

When trying to convince a politician, my rule is to focus on the people affected by the issue. In this case, that meant I had to tell the story of the clerks. I had to bring them to life not as bad, uncaring people, but as mostly young, not very well educated low-wage earners struggling to get by, often rushed, worried about their families, facing a line of people, wanting to serve them and to do a good job. They don't want to get into an argument. It's easier for them to just sell the cigarettes instead of asking for ID. I had to talk about the sting and ask the question, "What good did it do anyone to lock up a clerk or fine them?"

Then I proposed an easier, better way to keep tobacco products from the kids. Make everybody show an ID. Put the burden on the buyer. If kids are faking their age, arrest them, not the clerk. You will always make your case more powerful when you show a politician a real problem affecting real people in their district and give them a solution.

Checklist For Meeting With Your Elected Official.

1. Get clear in your own mind about what you want to achieve. Usually you will be visiting as part of a coordinated effort through your association. You will have an issue and information about the issue to bring to their attention. Your association should have given you a specific assignment such as:

- Present information and ask for a response or ask for support of a particular bill or concept.

- Get your targeted elected official to contact another elected official and ask for action, such as a vote in committee.

- Become a co-sponsor.

If you cannot say precisely what you want from this meeting, ask the question: Why are we doing this? If you cannot come up with an answer, maybe you shouldn't have a meeting.

2. Make an appointment. If the association has made your appointment, confirm it. If not, call the office where you are meeting and ask for the appointments secretary or scheduler. She may want to know in detail what you want to talk about, so be prepared to explain. Think of it as practice pitching your story. It's okay to lay your cards on the table early, since no one in politics likes surprises.

3. Follow up. When you get an appointment, follow up with a confirmation letter and send a copy to headquarters.

4. Inform yourself before the meeting. Gather biographical information on your targeted elected official. The more you know about the person, the better you can relate to them. Association staff may provide you with extensive, detailed information.

If you haven't received it, ask for it. You can get what you need from the Internet, either from the elected official's site, newspaper archives or just a general search.

It's a good idea to learn to do this on your own and to keep an eye out for information on TV and in newspapers back home. You only have one or two politicians to track and your association staff would have to monitor the whole Congress.

Get names of staffers you may encounter, their job titles and backgrounds. Get directions to the office and the office phone number in case you get lost. Make sure someone in your party has a cell phone.

5. Help the elected official and staff prepare for your meeting. Call and ask who is handling your issue. Send information that supports your case, as much as you wish, with an executive summary no longer than one page. (A staffer told me no one in Washington had read anything longer than one page since the typewriter was invented.) State what you want, why you want it and what it means to the district and to you personally.

In a follow-up call, ask if they need any more information and give them permission to call you any time at home or at the office.

6. Prepare yourself. Get your organization's issue paper and review it. However, keep in mind that nobody expects you to be an expert on legislation. Your job is to be the expert on your little piece of the issue as it affects you. If you can give the broader picture, that helps. But your priority is to tell your elected representative how your issue plays out in the district, in your practice and community and in your life. You are an expert on what's going on and that's what they need to hear from you.

7. Be informed. Find out what position your targeted senator or representative has taken on your issue in the past. Has this issue or anything similar come up in committee or for any kind of vote?

8. Know the process. Find out what the next step is in the legislative process (introduce the bill, committee hearing, mark up, etc.). Your professional lobbyist will know. Your targeted elected official may not know where your issue is in the legislative treadmill, and he will probably ask you. You can also avoid the embarrassment of learning that your bill has already been passed or defeated.

9. Bring notes. Take an index card and write down what you want from the elected official, as specifically as possible. Put down three or four reasons why the issue is important in the district and in your business. What is happening or will happen to real people in a general sense?

Picture a specific person who is being or will be affected. Jot down key words to remind yourself how this person will be affected. Be able to make this person come alive with a name, age, job, address, and so on. The story about a real person will be what they remember most of the time.

10. Get ready for culture shock. The staff you will encounter in the legislature and Congress may be younger than you and of a different outlook and ethnic background than the people you normally deal with.

Especially in Washington DC, you may find yourself sitting down with a twenty-something wearing baggy clothes who looks too young to be dealing with weighty matters. Avoid displaying shock or commenting on her age. (One of my clients came out of a series of meetings and said, "My God, the country is being run by children." It's true.) Regardless of her youth and inexperience, this person is in a position to help or hurt you. Speak with respect in a businesslike manner.

11. Take two other people. Although there may be internal reasons that force you to take more or less, taking too many people is the most common mistake people make, according to staff and elected officials. (I have had some express surprise that so many people came all this way, so maybe numbers do count sometimes.) Among other things, you will often be in a tiny, cramped space that has difficulty accommodating even three, especially in state offices. No matter how many you have, assign the following functions.

Presenter: Delivers the message and asks for help. Does most of the talking, working from 4 x 6 card or other notes. Keeps conversation on track and focuses on purpose of meeting. Has practiced and rehearsed the message. Stays on message and gets back on message.

Secretary: Handles papers, hands over background material as needed, gives a list of volunteer advocates who are present with names, employer (if relevant), mailing address (home), and phone numbers. Business cards are okay, but put your home phone number on them. If you use business cards, gather them before the meeting and hand them over in one stack all at once (no fumbling through purses and billfolds).

Observer: Takes notes of what is said, any requests for more information, promises made.

If the staffer says she will get back to you, ask when and let her know you are writing it down. You have a right to expect a prompt follow-up. Good notes equal power. Don't worry that staff will feel offended somehow.

This is a business meeting. If you feel the need to explain, just say, "We want to make sure we follow up on everything."

Look at body language and facial expressions of the targeted elected official and staff. Are they fidgeting, looking at watches, answering the phone? Are they merely polite or genuinely interested? Was the meeting ended with a pre-planned interruption such as a phone call? What was the tone of the meeting?

These things may tell you more than the words spoken. Watch to see if the listener really understands what is being said. It's not only okay but important to interrupt and suggest going back over something to make sure it is clear. Notice what kind of notes the staff and/or elected official are taking. Some are compulsive and take reams of notes. It always concerns me that they may not be listening, that perhaps the note taking is for show.

So I like to let them know up front that we will be giving them complete written information on everything we have to say. Frankly, I would rather have them listening and not taking so many notes.

I was once with a lawn care group talking to a member of Congress when they delivered what for them was a central article of faith about chemicals on lawns: "The dose is the poison." To the people in the industry, this was like saying "Do unto others..."

But the Congressman didn't move. I interrupted and said, "Congressman, they just said something important and I wonder if they made it clear?" He said he didn't know what it meant. We were able to back up and run it by him again with explanation. At the end of the meeting he had the central points we had come there to make.

12. At the meeting, take care of business. This is not a social gathering – it's a business meeting, very much like a sales call. While you don't want to be brusque, you do want to use your limited time well, which is another reason to keep the group small. Introductions take a long time and everyone may feel they have to chat or contribute. They don't. While you want to follow the lead of the person you are talking with, remember you have a purpose and an agenda. Say hello, give a brief introduction and a list of who is there with biographical information, and get to work. State what you want and why you want it.

13. Be observant. When you get a signal that your time is up, say, "Let me check my notes to make sure I said everything I came here to say." Then pause carefully. Look at your 4 x 6 card and think, "Did I ask for what I wanted?" Make sure you haven't missed anything. If you need to, restate your position and ask for what you want.

14. Be direct. Ask the staffer something like this: "When will you speak to Representative Smith and let him know what we said?" You might give the staffer a personal note with your home phone number and say, "Will you give this to her? Since we haven't been able to talk in person, I would like to talk by phone." Remember, one of the jobs of staff is to screen out people, to protect the elected official's time. You need to be assertive in showing that you want to speak with your elected official, if not now, then soon. I have had staffers tell me that sometimes they just take information and file it away. This is not what you want.

15. Follow up again. Send a note of thanks to all concerned, including the relevant staff, receptionists and so on. Briefly reiterate what you and your observer heard in the way of results. Thank them for support or urge reconsideration as appropriate and assure them that any promised follow-up will be coming soon.

16. Call or send a report to your association headquarters. This increases the value of your meeting many times and helps your lobbyist plan strategy.

Two tips: First, never threaten or use language that can be interpreted as threatening. Statements such as, "We helped you get elected last time," "We have a lot of voters in our organization," or "This will get a lot of votes," will make your politician defensive and turn him off immediately.

Anyone in office already knows the political reality. Not only is it unnecessary, but it will also be regarded as crude, rude and amateurish. If you have the power to intimidate, you do not need to say so; your politician already knows it. If you don't have it, you will look foolish.

Second, communicate with a purpose. Some people call or write so often and about so many topics they are considered slightly daffy and lonely. "Don't be a pen pal," said one staffer. Writing about every topic that strikes your fancy will turn you into a pen pal wannabe. These letters are considered pitiful and irritating.

I am often asked how many times you can communicate. I think as long as you have something new to say, it's okay. But just repeating the same stuff quickly becomes an irritating nag and is counterproductive. My gut feeling is that you need to be in front of staff and politicians with something useful and/or helpful or in person four to six times a year just to be remembered.

In all of this I urge you to remember the concept advanced by John Naisbitt in his pioneering book "Megatrends."

He called it high-tech/high touch. What he meant was that the more we use technology to communicate, the more impersonal it gets and the more we crave "touching." Big-screen TVs haven't killed the movies because people want a shared experience. People still want to go to the office even though they could do most of their work from any computer in the world.

Politicians particularly crave real human interaction because they are among the most people-people of all. They, and their offices, are responding more and more to high-tech communications by screening them out and focusing on the high-touch personal communications.

If you doubt this, send an email and see what happens.

Becoming A Human With High Touch Value

One of the most effective leave-behinds I've seen was created by Chuck Johnson of Farwell, Mich. Chuck is an avid motorcyclist. He had been trying to get to see Sen. Debbie Stabenow (D-MI) without success. He thought it might be that she didn't have time to talk with a "biker."

Motorcyclists, or bikers, often have an image problem with people and politicians who don't know them. So Chuck created an 8 ½" x 11" bound booklet to leave with members of Congress. It contained his resume and color photos.

The first page told about himself in considerable detail in resume format.

Then he had pictures of his wife, a Methodist minister, in her clerical robes standing beside the church sign. Next were pictures of him on his motorcycle, with his grandchildren, and finally of himself on the motorcycle in a parade with a huge yellow man-size chicken character on the back – the sort of mascot you see at a football game. The parade kicks off an annual chicken barbecue in Farwell.

Cutting Through The Clutter

Chuck reports that a staffer gave this handout to the senator, probably with some amazement. Senator Stabenow thumbed through it and realized that she had walked in that parade and seen the chicken character and Chuck. She got in touch with him and he was finally able to talk with her.

He had made a personal connection.

I don't know what's going to work for you. But I do know it is important that you become something more than just a title or a business card. Some people do this well just by telling about themselves. The important step is to help the people you talk with remember you as a multidimensional person who is part of the community.

You're not just a doctor, nurse, coder or medical practice manager. You have family, activities and other connections that make you part of the community. In explaining this, you may find some common bond with the person you are talking with. At the very least, you become more memorable.

Money: A Moral, Ethical, Legal, and Effective Tool to Achieve Your Goals

Many people feel awkward and uneasy about money and politics.

You may have read in the newspaper and seen on TV how political action committees influence members of Congress, how people with the biggest PACs seem to get what they want, how money can determine who gets elected and that the PACs have the money. You've seen lobbyists and members of Congress go to jail. You may have reacted with stunned disbelief at the representative with $90,000 in his freezer. It looks like something you don't want to be part of.

Whatever your feelings, it's important to understand that money does have a role in politics and to see how it is used – both what it can and cannot do.

As you consider money and politics, ask this question: Do you want to work within the system or try to change it? If you want to change the system, you will have a lot of company among professional lobbyists and corporate and association executives. Many find the practice of raising and distributing money distasteful. Many people in Congress and the states want to change the way we finance elections.

The problem is, no one has been able to come up with a better way that people will support. Given that it costs a lot of money to communicate to voters and we want to have elections, a lot of money has to be raised from somewhere. Quite a few state house and senate races are now costing more than $1 million. Few people can afford that, so candidates have to raise money wherever they can.

You can make a strong case for publicly financing elections. For $10 to $50 per citizen, depending on how much reform you want to buy, we could pay for elections. But not enough people want to do that, so what we have is a system of privatized elections. It's almost like raising money in the stock market.

Candidates have to make the case and persuade people to invest in something they believe in. So in a very real sense, the system makes sure only people with support can run.

By contrast, we pay for police, fire and health departments; we pay for juries, judges and prosecutors; we even pay senators, representatives, governors and presidents, once they are elected. But to get elected, they have to beg and borrow from people whose main interest is getting something in return. Don't blame the people who run for office or the people who give them money for behaving the way they do. All of us are operating in the system taxpayers could change tomorrow, if they wanted to.

Whatever you think, my goal is to help you work within the system. Incidentally, these techniques can help you change the system, if that's what you want.

Political Action Committees ARE The Reform

It's good to remember that political action committees (PACs) are the reform. They were created by Congress and the states to shine light on the flow of money into campaigns. By and large it has worked. We have a system of campaign finance that is transparent and honest. It used to be much worse.

I had a conversation with a retired banker from Georgia a few years back. He told me part of his job had been to act as the political "bagman." He took the gym bags full of cash over to the capitol in Atlanta. He did not actually go into the governor's office; he went off to the side. One of the staff people would take the bag and thank him. He said he had delivered as much as $50,000 in cash at a time – many times – this way.

The record is clear that influence used to be bought that way, with cash passed under the table. In the case of Georgia senator Herman Talmadge, persons unknown to him used to put large bills in his suit coat pockets, much to his amazement. I'm not saying it doesn't happen anymore, but it's a lot cleaner than it used to be and the PAC system is the reason.

PAC money is honest, legal money, reported and on the record, and those records are available for anyone to look at. For now, money to run campaigns will continue to come mostly from individuals writing private checks, whether to politicians directly or to PACs. (Some states allow corporate contributions, and, interestingly, they don't seem to have any better or worse government than the others. But that's another story.)

The major objection many people have is that a PAC contribution feels like an attempt to buy a vote. Having talked to hundreds of PAC money recipients, both state and federal, and to the people who give out the money, I don't think you can buy a vote – at least not with PAC money, which is in the public record.

I did have one politician say in a public meeting that the money does influence his thinking. He said it is a lot easier to vote with the people who have given money than those who haven't.

His comments affirm what I have said: that many times politicians don't really care which way an issue goes, and it really doesn't matter that much to the public interest, so they vote with their friends. I respect his candor, and I suspect that is true for all elected officials.

Are You Buying Votes With PAC Money?

However, I still say PAC money cannot buy a vote for a couple of important reasons. One is very practical: The limits on PAC contributions mean that even if a vote were for sale, you couldn't give enough through a PAC.

Another reason is that, in all probability, your opponents have given money to the same people you have. Generally speaking, all the players engaged are giving money and the money tends to balance out or cancel out. This brings up another important reason to give! If your opponents are giving and you aren't, who cares more about the issue and about the elected official?

Reasons To Give to Your PAC

The PAC is the most efficient and effective way to raise campaign money from a wide base of contributors. It's an efficient and effective way to make your voice heard in the legislature and Congress. In fact, it is very hard to present a credible political presence without a PAC. If you have no PAC, you may not be taken seriously. You just don't look like a serious organization. If you want to be heard, it helps to have a PAC.

Here are some reasons why PACs are effective:

1. Working together, we have more impact than all of us working separately. The money we give is pooled so it has more impact. Former senator David Boren of Oklahoma once pointed out when opposing PACs that the average U.S. senator must raise $13,000 a week for six years to finance the next election. (The number is higher today.)

"If people come in to see you and one is a student and one is a small businessman and one is a teacher and one is a farmer and one is a PAC person with big campaign contributions, who are you going to see in your limited time?" he asked.

Of course, the answer is that many of those farmers and teachers and small business people had contributed personally and to a PAC. Some of us, when we give money to candidates, will give $100, $250 or maybe $500. But a contribution of that size is rare. Most people will give less than $100. Candidates value those and like to brag that they are getting lots of small contributions.

With the advent of the Internet, raising enough small contributions to fund a campaign may become possible at the national or presidential level. But while candidates love to get those small contributions, they are expensive to recruit; they can't remember the contributors and don't even know who they are.

Therefore, the key to influential giving is to give enough to rise out of the herd and get noticed.

By pulling together those small contributions into a large PAC check from your association, you can have a major impact and your association will be remembered and appreciated.

2. Unlike most of us who only pay attention to politics during the election campaigns, the PAC is eternally vigilant. It keeps an eye on elected officials and issues all year round, and can take action as needed and keep you informed.

3. The PAC allows us to hold elected officials accountable. If they don't support us, we won't support them. We may support their opponent. There is a subtle but real effect on politicians when they know you have a huge war chest you can throw into elections or issue fights. Usually they would like to avoid a fight, and certainly an expensive one. The thought that you might go public and oppose them can have a powerful deterrent effect.

One political operative told me this story: There was a member of Congress from Pennsylvania who consistently opposed his union clients on an issue involving the National Labor Relations Board. Finally they decided they had to do something serious to get the Congressman to change his position. They prepared a series of radio ads to run in the district explaining the Congressman's stand and the effect on people in the district (from the union's point of view, of course).

They went to the Congressman and told him they didn't want to run the ads and they didn't want to get into a fight, but they were prepared to if he couldn't compromise. They played the ads for him. He blinked. Rather than get into a fight with a well-financed opponent, he cut a deal. Having a well-stocked PAC is like having missiles in a silo: You may never have to fire them to get the benefit.

4. PAC money has more impact because it is easier to get. Candidates have to spend money to raise money from individuals, but PAC money comes in large lump sums. Unless you are Howard Dean or some other famous politician, it's almost impossible to run a campaign on money raised in $25 and $50 contributions. It's too expensive to get each one and you use all your money raising money.

5. PAC contributions give candidates a clear idea of where you stand on the issue. When you give personal money, usually the only thing they know is that you like them personally. A personal contribution may be misunderstood. The PAC money represents a specific interest, not just an individual. That interest – or rather its PAC – has carefully considered which candidates to support. That interest group is permanent; it was here last year and it'll be here next year, as will the possibility of support or opposition.

6. The PAC expands your influence beyond your own political district. It directs your money to candidates you may not know about throughout the state and nation who need your support. I seldom encounter a person who sends a personal check to a distant district, to a candidate for whom he cannot vote, unless it's someone running for president.

What if the person running for office from your district is adamantly opposed to your interest? Or just doesn't care? Or is weak and can't help?

You won't give, but how can you identify those people who support your views? The PAC knows. The PAC looks around the whole state and nation and applies your money where it will do the most good.

7. The PAC makes a carefully studied, well-informed decision on whom to support. Many things go on in Congress and the legislature that people outside the process don't know about. The PAC and your lobbyists support and oppose candidates based on inside knowledge of what really happened to your issues.

This differs significantly from the way personal donations are decided. Givers often don't know much about a candidate's voting record or competency in matters that don't show up in votes. My experience has been that the most important factor in whether people contribute personal money is whether they know and like a candidate.

Most people simply don't have the time or interest to focus on what our elected officials do in office. We don't know all the different ways and occasions they may have acted for or against our interest.

One state representative in Florida told this story to a group of Realtors I was training. He explained that he was a banker and served on several committees relating to banking and finance. Having been there some years, he carried a lot of clout. The Realtors had supported him and he considered himself their friend.

The Realtors were supporting a bill that came up in one of his committees that related to finance. Although he had some reservations about the bill, they weren't serious, and so, because of his friendship, he said nothing. "I could have killed that bill, but I sat on my hands," he said. His point was that this action – or inaction – was not something that would show up in voting records, but it was important.

Most of us are unlikely to know about such actions and unlikely to support someone far from our home district who helps us this way. But the PAC knows.

8. The PAC makes its decisions based only on your issues as decided by the membership and leadership of your association. Sometimes it will support a candidate that some members don't like because of her stand on unrelated issues. That's because the PAC is designed to support only narrow issues.

Maybe she is a Democrat and you are a Republican. Your personal feelings on those issues may not allow you to give money to that candidate. But that same candidate may have consistently supported budget increases and other issues that help you.

The PAC will make a cold, calculated investment to protect your interest, one you might not make because of the conflicting issues. The PACs I work with that are most successful operate systematically and dispassionately to evaluate candidates.

You have a local and perhaps a state and national committee that considers candidates and elected officials already in office. They go through a rigorous process of evaluating what candidates have said and done, their electability and their understanding of issues.

They try hard to separate out the stands on social issues, political parties, and other factors not relevant to the narrow focus of the organization.

They ask, "Which candidate is best for this special interest?" and then invest your money where it will represent you the best.

9. PACs are legally established by the legislature and Congress. The purpose is to establish an open, honest regulated system by which people can join together to support or oppose candidates. The PAC system allows the public to know who contributes and who receives money. PACs are one way we have chosen to finance elections.

10. The PAC is an important education device for elected officials. Properly done, the process by which your association decides who will get PAC money becomes an important communication medium to elected officials. I learned this when I ran for state house of representatives in my home state of North Carolina. Only one PAC was interested in my race. It was a coalition of builders, Realtors, apartment companies and developers.

They sent around a person who lived and worked in my district with a long questionnaire. On the surface, the purpose was to find out how I felt about the issues they were concerned with.

It was a real eye-opener for me. I had no idea how to answer many of the questions, although it was clear I needed to know the answers if I were to be effective after I was elected. In answering their questions, I had to ask for more information and think hard about what I heard. It was an introduction to a lot of issues and information I had never had access to.

When I set up PAC committees for my clients, I recommend a formal process in which a committee screens all candidates. This way you get a dialogue between the committee and the candidates. When candidates are appealing for money from your PAC, they will learn about your association and your issues better than at any other time.

11. Your PAC is an important tool to protect your specific interest. It is designed and operates to protect your business and create a positive, profitable climate. When you think about whether to give and how much, ask yourself, "What is it worth to get the results I want?"

People in oil marketing, banking, logging, fishing and many other industries have awakened to find their ability to stay in business compromised by a failure to pay attention to the political climate they operate in. The same thing can happen to issues you care about. Giving to your PAC makes sure someone is looking after you and your interest.

Former Wyoming Senator Alan Simpson was talking about grassroots involvement, but he summed it up well when he said, "Take part or get taken apart."

Other Ways To Give And Be Noticed

It is also important to write personal checks and hand them to a politician whenever possible, even if they are small. You get about the same benefit from showing up at fundraisers such as barbecues just to be seen (and eat and drink).

Organizing a home-based fundraiser can be the most powerful relationship builder of all. Although I call it "home-based," you can do it in an office or hotel or wherever. You just pay for food and drink and ask your friends to attend and bring a check.

You or your spouse may have done this for a church, school or charity such as a heart association.

The same process works for politicians and you may get much more return on your investment.

The Most Powerful System: Key Contacts

The most successful advocacy organizations have adopted a "key contact" (KC) grassroots system: the association selects a member who lives and works in the district (or state for U.S. senators) to be the key contact. This is someone willing to build a supportive, trusting relationship and deliver the association's message as needed.

This contrasts with broad-based (BB) systems in which the association has a list of names and sends action alerts to everyone. The difference is significant.

Most organizations that think they have a grassroots operation have only a database of names. They have no idea when people communicate or how effectively. Even organizations that use Internet systems, and there are plenty of good ones, often aren't much better off even though they can track the communications.

Yes, I know Howard Dean energized a great many people. I know MoveOn.org has mobilized millions. I know Obama has a zillion email addresses. But your issues are not the same and will not be resolved the same way. Nor do you have the capacity to mobilize tens of thousands of people. You don't need to. Look at the difference from a politician's viewpoint:

Key Contact: Message comes from a known, trusted person
Broad based: Message from unknowns, perhaps faked

KC: Often delivered face-to-face
BB: Usually e-mail, easily dismissed, ignored, and discounted

KC: Message detailed, tailored to the person and the moment
BB: Message is repetitious, canned, minimal, simplistic

KC: Depends on persuasion, logic, mutual benefit

BB: Depends on volume

KC: Provides two-way communication, feedback and response
BB: One-way or with only form letters exchanged

KC: Focused, efficient, targets only specific decision makers
BB: Shotgun, hit or miss, wastes effort

KC: Politicians and staff appreciate input from constituents
BB: Mass campaigns cause problems and are resented

KC: Committed person willing to invest time and energy
BB: Minimal investment in e-mail means minimal concern

A key contact system will serve you and your association best. It is a system, an organization, a campaign, not just a list. It is action versus hope. It is accountability versus guesswork. A key contact system is based on these concepts:

- Recruit, train and support specific people to build long-term relationships with politicians

- Maximize effort by targeting key decision makers in Congress and the legislature first and foremost Support those politicians personally and organizationally with help of many kinds, especially money

When setting up a key contact system, it's a good idea to spell out your expectations in writing or else people will create their own. In that case, they may perceive the job to be much more or much less than you actually want.

Here's a sample job description adapted from associations I have worked with. It tells you what is usually expected of a key contact. If your organization doesn't have a job description for volunteer advocates, this will help you develop one.

Association Key
Contact Job Description

General Responsibilities:

Key contact agrees to build and maintain strong, positive relationships with assigned members of the United States Senate and House of Representatives and contact them as requested and deliver PAC check.

Specific Objectives:

Key contact is responsible for staying abreast of association legislative priorities and initiatives through association government relations mailings, Internet postings, and the newsletter.

Key contact is to meet personally with a designated legislator at least two times a year to review priority legislative issues.

Key contact is to invite legislator to visit business for information session and photo op at least annually.

Key contact is to deliver PAC campaign check to assigned legislator as necessary.

Key contact is to attend local meetings with association staff as needed. This includes attendance at the annual association government relations summer group meetings and probably local political meetings the assigned legislator attends.

Communicating Issues:

Key contact is to respond to requests for contact as indicated in legislative alerts. Action requested may consist of writing a letter, coordinating a letter-writing campaign, making a personal visit, or calling a legislator.

Reporting:

Key contact is to promptly report back to government relations staff (by faxing the response form, e-mail, or telephone) on contacts made; report should include any legislator comments on issues discussed.

Key contact is expected to participate in political action committee with a leadership contribution, personal contribution, and volunteer time.

How You Gonna Call? Effectiveness Rating Chart For Communicating With Elected Officials

100   Eyeball–to-eyeball. It's hard to say "no" when you're looking someone in the eye.

98   Personal letter (your own words, localized to the official's district with a hand-written note)

93   Thoughtful phone call with dialogue

80   Fax (personalized)

80   Meeting with senior staff

50   E-mail, if they know you

40   Phone call with instructions to vote "yes" or "no," leaving your name, which they may or may not recognize.

40   Meeting with junior staff

30   Obviously orchestrated impersonal communication in any form (gang phone calls from a convention, stimulated form telegrams, e-mails, faxes, etc., even with names of individuals in the district)

20   E-mail, if they don't know you

15   Preprinted anything (form letter, post card, issue paper, fax)

10   Petitions (no matter how many signatures)

0   Anything from outside the district, unless you represent a national or state organization with people in the district or are communicating to a committee chair or committee staff, in which

case it could go as high as 80

Members of Congress and state legislatures are buried in mail, phone calls, faxes, and e-mail they will never see. They barely have enough staff to handle all the stuff that comes in, much less give it consideration. If you look at congressional websites, they all tell you to communicate only with your own elected official – the one you can vote for.

So focus on and multiply things we know have maximum impact. Personal, eyeball-to-eyeball relationships followed up and reinforced by thoughtful, permanent written communication are about the only things that can penetrate the tidal wave of messages flowing into politicians' offices.

One chief of staff from a Washington office told me his Congresswoman sometimes meets with twenty people in a day. On top of all the other work members do, can you imagine how hard it is to remember any of this?

That's why your relationship with the politician and staff is probably the most important determinant whether you get a response. If you doubt that, here is a list compiled by Bill Posey, who served in the Florida House of Representatives and then in the state senate. He's now in the U.S. House of Representatives.

His district includes part of Walt Disney World and all of Cape Canaveral. He is a good example of how building a relationship early, when a politician first gets started, can pay off long term. I would not be surprised to see him in the U.S. Senate some day.

Posey's Practical Pointers For Grass Roots Lobbying

1 point minimum impact; 10 points maximum impact

1 point Send photocopied letters

2 points Send out faxes on hot issues

3 points Send copy of monthly magazine or newsletter

4 points Call the legislative office

5 points Send personal letters, regardless of quality

2 to 8 points Publicize high ratings or awards depending
 upon quality and prestige

-2 points Call them at their regular/real job about legislation

-5 points Call them at home

-10 points Call them at home late at night

Meet personally by appointment to discuss positions and issues:

10 points If you are a voter in the district

10 points more If you are a contributor

10 points more If you are both

1 point If you supported the opponent and it was a nasty campaign (stay away until you are in a position to offer support next time)

When discussing business over dinner, use the opportunity to build relationships (in most cases, 1,000 lobster dinners won't buy support for your issues, regardless of what the press says).

Author's note: I respect Bill and he has graciously appeared in several seminars and impressed the audiences with his forthrightness. However, I differ with him on one item. I think it is usually a waste of time to routinely send newsletters to politicians.

Can you imagine how many people send monthly newsletters to politicians? They don't have time to read all the stuff they want to much less your junk mail. They only need to hear from you when you have something specific to say.

If you have something in a newsletter that merits attention, like a picture of the politician, send it with a letter, opened to the right page with the item of interest circled in red ink.

Seven Steps For Creating A Powerful In-Person Encounter

Checklist For Delivering Your Message

When you visit an elected official, certain things will increase your effectiveness. This is a seven-step checklist for a successful meeting.

1. Tell them who you are: Don't just state your name and title; also tell a little about yourself, your business, your personal history and your family. You want them to know you as a human being, not just an issue advocate. Make sure he knows you represent an association, not just yourself, so he connects your visit to your professional lobbyist.

2. Anecdote/story: Bring your issue to life in human terms. Tell about real patients and situations from the politician's state or district who are or will be affected. Think "soap opera" with details, names, dates and places; make it come alive.

3. What you want: Make sure the politician knows exactly what you came for: vote yes, vote no, co-sponsor, speak to someone on the committee-, and so on.

4. Why it's a good idea: Have at least three sound reasons why this elected official should support your position, especially focusing on the impact in his state or district.

5. Ask for support: Look directly in his eyes, lock on and ask, "Will you vote with us (write the letter, co-sponsor or whatever)?"

6. Remember thank-you notes: Send handwritten notes to everyone you talk with.

7. Report results: Always detail the results of the meeting back to the headquarters of your association.

Communications That Work

The single most powerful weapon in your political arsenal is a letter. Not just any letter, but a special sort of letter. Given the security measures in place, sending postal mail is no longer a good option for Congress, so "letter" includes fax and e-mail.

But sending something that looks like an ordinary e-mail will cause your communication to be discounted by many people in Congress. So think about sending a PDF document that looks like letterhead and contains an ink-like signature. It may be printed and given to the member of Congress to carry outside the office, read on the plane and so on. You can also use html to create an e-mail that looks like letterhead.

However, many offices are wary of opening attachments, so e-mail and faxes are your best option. Whatever you do, realize that appearances are part of the message and ordinary e-mails make less of an impression than something more businesslike. It is likely your message will be printed out, filed and read off line.

Considering all I've said about how elected officials want to hear from their constituents, I strongly recommend you indicate you are one up front. This means in the subject line of an e-mail and the first line of an e-mail, fax or letter, you say something like, "I live in District [XX]," giving the correct number for the district your official serves. For the U.S. Senate, "I live in [City] and [State]."

If there is any way, make a personal connection. "You probably don't remember, but we shook hands at the barbecue last August in Des Moines."

Why write? Letters take more effort than a phone call and require you to get your thoughts in order. They are permanent. They can be copied. They go into files by issue. They are hard to ignore.

As you set out to influence your government, put it in writing. As you write, remember that to be special your letter must be thoughtful and personal. That is not to say that form letters don't have any impact. They do. When enough people send in letters saying essentially the same thing, using the same words, elected officials know they are part of an organized campaign. The fact that they know it's organized is not only okay, it's necessary. You need to be part of something larger than one person to get attention.

However, to truly change the mind or vote of an elected official, you need to appeal not only to their political instincts but also to their reason and emotion. They are interested in who is touched by your issue and how they are affected. How will it play out for their constituents?

They are interested in who cares, how much you care and why you care. They are interested in whether you know what you are talking about and have anything worthwhile to say. Consider the following letter (name omitted).

This was given to me, proudly, by a nursing home administrator.

Read it and see what you think the politician's reaction would be.

Re: $29 million cut in Medicaid
Dear Governor,

Apparently, sir, you have forgotten that the elderly in today's Florida nursing homes are those citizens who just a few years ago either fought, farmed, worked in industries, paid dearly for lost loved ones and paid taxes for World War I, II, Korea, and Vietnam. After the world wars, they paid for our hospitals, constructed universities, built interstates, fed other nations, and are directly responsible for all these contributions to the greatest nation that exists.

Today, after their strength has been spent and finances exhausted, they live hopelessly with their last days at the mercy of unappreciative politicians.

How can elected officials conscientiously live with themselves and their conscience, day after day spending billions after billions of American dollars for projects all over the world and failing to provide adequate funds for our own?

Cuts of $29 million, plus no increase in Medicaid rates for the care of Florida's infirm elderly, are absolutely uncalled for. Governor, you can do better.

The next few months will tell all Floridians if you are a responsible person, the man who supports the health and welfare of the elderly, sick, and infirm, or just another heartless politician.

As a lifetime Democrat, I pray that you will come to your senses and act responsibly.

Sincerely,
John Doe

At first glance, many people like this letter. However, consider the tone.

What does this writer think about politicians and about the governor? What is the governor likely to remember from this letter? Would a staff person pass this on to the governor? If the governor did see this, I suspect the words "heartless politician" may hang heavy in his mind. I also suspect the governor does not see himself as a "heartless politician."

The only reason this letter gives him to change his mind is that one slightly upset person will think he's heartless. It is personal, but is it thoughtful? Does it cause the reader to stop and think? A letter needs to give specific reasons to support your position, just like an in-person meeting.

For example, what if the writer had said:

I'm writing to urge you to restore the $29 million in proposed Medicaid cuts. I realize you face tough choices in balancing the state budget. But I am worried that if the funds for Medicaid are cut further, the steps we will have to take to economize on the cost of care will be harmful to our elderly nursing home residents.

I've been an administrator for twenty-seven years. In my nursing home we are certified for 150 beds and usually they are all filled. The state pays us $88 a day to give near-hospital-level care to elderly residents. While we will always find ways to provide adequate care, if you cut the already meager funding we have, we will have to consider cutting some things that make a major difference in the quality of life our elderly enjoy. For example, under your proposed budget we have to consider cutting:

- Trips to the mall for our mobile elderly. We take them once a week and for many it is their only contact with the outside world other than television.

- Premium canned beans. We can cut back by using the canned beans with ends in them, although they often cause problems for elderly with dentures.

- Staff. We have more aides on duty than the state requires because when an old person wants a drink of water, we want him or her to be able to get it promptly. At state minimums, an aide may care for ten residents and just can't get to them often enough.

There is more, and I invite you to come to our nursing home and see for yourself. We provide excellent care on the funds we receive, and in fact, nursing homes provide the most efficient and cost-effective care of any institutions in the state. But we are in danger of falling back to merely adequate custodial care because of rising expenses and reduced funding.

The proposed budget cuts of $29 million in Medicaid will substantially reduce the quality of life for our elderly in nursing homes. I hope you will look carefully for other ways to balance the budget and restore the cuts as proposed by the Southern Association of Nursing Homes.

Please let me know your feelings about this as soon as possible. If you want more information, I will be glad to provide it.

This version is designed to show sympathy for the governor, who has to make tough choices, and to give enough specifics to show the effect of budget cuts. The beans, the mall trip, the glass of water – all are designed to conjure up specific images. They are real examples given to me when I questioned nursing home administrators about what would happen if the Medicaid budget were cut.

Which letter do you think would have a more positive impact?

The second letter mentions the association, so the governor knows the letter is part of a widespread campaign. Notice it also tells something of the experience and position of the writer. Remember, you are an expert in your area. It's important to let the elected official know you are knowledgeable.

Enough letters like this, thoughtful and personal, to governors and legislators or the resident and members of Congress, can have dramatic effect.

It helps if you let the recipient know you are politically savvy. Tell them what you want, where your issue is in the process, when the next action step is likely and what the effect is on real people in your business and community.

Keep it short. One page is usually enough. If you have more to say, put it in another letter and send it later. If you don't get a reply within ten days, call and ask what happened to your letter. You may have to send it again.

But don't quit until you get an answer.

If you get an answer and don't like it, write again and ask for a conversation, saying this issue is really important to you.

AND YET...

Over the years I have said, and almost everyone else in the business has said, a one-page letter is best. That's certainly true if you are trying to show that you, someone known and respected, is taking a stand. But I'm not sure that one page is best if you are trying to persuade someone to change his or her mind.

My thinking on this started to change while I was standing in the office of Texas State Rep. Patricia Gray with some folks from her district. As we talked, she noticed the name tag of a man with us and said, "You sent me a letter, didn't you?" She explained that she had not responded yet because she was still thinking about the issues raised in the letter.

In my mind, the fact she remembered it and was thinking about it was significant. She was chair of the Sunset Commission, which was reviewing laws to decide which should be retained, changed or eliminated. I was so struck by the moment I got permission to reprint the following exchange of letters. First, the one to her:

The Honorable Patricia Gray
Texas House of Representatives
P.O. Box 2910
Austin, Texas 78769

Dear Representative Gray:

The Texas Credit Union Commission is going through the Sunset review process this session. There are various proposals to change the agency's governance and renewal term. I believe the proposals would be adverse to the agency's effectiveness because they emanate from the interests of banking groups.

The banking industry is engaged in an aggressive campaign to thwart the ongoing development and success of credit unions.

Please consider that the Credit Union Commission has been an effective regulatory body since 1969. It should be renewed for another 12 years – not for only 4 years as urged by banking interests. Also, the commission's structure of 6 industry members and 3 public members has worked effectively since 1983 when the public members were added. That structure should be kept intact because it has proven to be effective.

Finally, there is a proposal to complicate the Commission's existing administrative procedures with burdensome hearings for handling matters, such as charter and bylaw amendments. These matters have been effectively and fairly administered in the past. Such unnecessary hearings would unduly hamper the orderly development of credit unions.

Please give careful consideration to these matters. We want to be able to continue giving good service to our members.

Sincerely
Roger McCrary
Chairman of the Board

This letter reads quickly, but it is a little longer than one page. It got the following response:

Dear Mr. McCrary,

Thank you for writing my office regarding your concerns for the Credit Union Commission. I am very supportive of the concept of credit unions and the invaluable service and access they provide to the community.

As you may know, on Tuesday, September 24, the Sunset Commission formally met to vote on the proposed recommendations affecting the structure of the Texas Credit Union Commission. The Sunset Commission voted to maintain the Credit Union Commission's autonomy; however, we recommended they comply with some public notice and comment before their hearings regarding approval or denial of charter applications, field membership expansion, and mergers.

The Sunset Commission also voted to improve the public's representation on the Credit Union Commission's Board, which is a policy that every state agency must comply with to ensure the public receives adequate input.

The Sunset Commission did not recommend consolidating the Credit Union Commission with the

Finance Commission, since the Finance Commission will not be reviewed by the Sunset Commission for possible restructuring until 2001.

I am frankly at a loss to understand how these two very mild changes will undermine credit unions in Texas. I respectfully disagree that all is completely rosy with the regulation of credit unions. The Sunset review found that one-quarter of the state-regulated credit unions had financial problems serious enough to warrant a remedial monitoring program. Only twenty of those improved enough to be removed from remedial monitoring by the end of the year assessed.

Once again, I appreciate your taking the time to write my office regarding your thoughts on the Credit Union Commission.

Sincerely,
Patricia Gray

I like this exchange, even though the writer did not get what he wanted. Representative Gray gave careful consideration to his letter but just disagreed. You can see in her letter that she had explored the issue carefully and had her facts in order.

Getting the politician to think is more than half the battle.

The other half is giving them something they will remember and that also comes from their district. Here is what I would consider to be an almost – as you will see – perfect letter.

This letter resulted from a conversation I had with a physician, Dr. Brendle Glomb, M.D., PCCP, FAAP, in Austin, Tex., who was coming to Washington with his professional association, The American College of Chest Physicians. We talked at length about what would work and as a result, he hand delivered this to his two senators and representative's offices and discussed the letter with staff.

Senator/Congressman:

I am a Pediatric Pulmonologist and pediatric critical care specialist and a voter in Austin. I live and vote in your district. I would like to take the opportunity to illustrate a point about Medicaid and its devaluation of patient care, especially pediatric care.

The attached paperwork represents two invoices, if you will. (He actually provided copies.) One invoice is a recent bill for my automobile. Circled and starred is the price per hour of my Goodyear mechanics time to work on my car. The other invoice is an EOB (Explanation of Benefits; "payment confirmation") from Medicaid for an hour of my time spent with a 5-year-old boy with severe, persistent asthma. Circled and starred is the price per hour that Medicaid decides my time is worth.

The notations for that visit were 4 pages long and encompassed all aspects of the patient's interim and past pulmonary history, physical examination, family history, assessment and medical plans for his future.

My mechanic, a man or woman I don't know and have never met, was paid $84 per hour for his time (or his shop). I trust that he/she is properly trained and has the experience to do a good job. I have no idea. I was reimbursed $37.34 for the hour of my time. I spent 10 years in post-graduate training to become a specialist. I have been in practice for more than 15 years. I have an established and trusted relationship with my patient and his family.

The little boy, prior to seeing me, was hospitalized eleven times in the preceding 12 months. Three of those hospitalizations involved the pediatric intensive care unit and, on one admission, he was intubated and placed on a ventilator for 3 days. The number of emergency room visits was in the dozens per year. The cost to Medicaid for a year of this young boy's care ran in the tens of thousands of dollars per year. Since being cared for by a Pediatric Pulmonary specialist, 6 months ago, he has not been re-hospitalized, has visited the ER only once (for a *broken arm), and sees me only quarterly, at similar or less expense to Medicaid per visit ($37.34).*

A cost analysis, done by an outside consultant, shows that our average Medicaid reimbursement, per patient contact, is minus $10, i.e., it costs our practice $10 to see each and every Medicaid patient. There is NO REIMBURSEMENT. Essentially, we are taxed for the "privilege."

For the first time in my career, we have been forced to limit the Medicaid load that we can accept in our office, due exclusively to the cost of doing business. Unfortunately, we are the ONLY Pediatric Pulmonary group in Central Texas. Medicaid children will go without specialist care.

Thank you for your time and consideration in this matter. I am happy to speak with you at anytime, at your convenience, about this and other healthcare issues related to both your Medicaid and private pay/insured constituents. I can be reached at the following numbers:

(He gave his home, office, cell and pager numbers.)

Sincerely,
Wm. Brendle Glomb, M.D.

So, great letter, right? What happened?

Nothing. About two months later I called to follow up and Dr. Glomb was disappointed and discouraged. So I took another look at the letter and the situation.

He had talked to very junior staff at each stop on the hill. He wondered if they understood what he was talking about.

The salutation, "senator/representative," may have made the letter look like a form letter. It might have had more impact if he had addressed it personally to the senators and representative by name.

This may be most important: The letter doesn't make the ask and neither did he. If offers to discuss, but does not say, "I want to talk with you about this" or "When can we get together?" It leaves the recipient free to do nothing. And that's what happened.

At our last discussion, we talked about these points and he agreed to fax his representative with a request for a discussion. My hunch is that this letter, good as it was, never got to a senior staff person or the members of Congress.

It may also be that they didn't want to do anything or, in the absence of the specific ask, didn't know what to do.

Part II
The PEOPLE

Front Line Providers:
They Make The Difference

Politics is all about the people who make our democracy work: politicians, lobbyists, advocates and staff. Professional lobbyists are the least understood and most maligned participants. In my own experience, they are almost all highly ethical people who believe deeply in the process. Sure, there are bad apples who break the law, just as there are in journalism, law and medicine.

But a lobbyists' only currency is their credibility and that, plus a host of disclosure laws and regulations, keep them at least as honest as any other profession.

The same is true of elected office holders, even though we get frequent examples of immorality, bribery and dishonesty.

No matter how discouraged you may get, or disgusted, at the behavior of the few, keep this in mind: If you drop out, you leave the field to your opponents.

Paula Szypko, M.D.

Paula Szypko, M.D., FCAP is the former Chair, College of American Pathologists Federal and State Affairs Committee. I met Paula Szypko when I did training at the pathologist lobby day in Washington DC She had been politically active for many years already.

In The Beginning

I was a busy pathologist, a mom, trying to have a life, when I got a call from the College of American Pathologists Washington office shortly after the 1994 election. They asked me to come to Washington and have what was called an interface session with my new Congressman, Representative Richard Burr. I said I'd be happy to, but actually because of the redistricting in North Carolina, I was no longer in his district.

I was surprised when I went to vote that his name wasn't the one on the ballot; it was someone else. They said, "Well Dr. Szypko, he doesn't need to know that, so why don't you come on anyhow," and I did, and that was the beginning.

The meeting started as a breakfast meeting, and ultimately I was set up to meet with him in his office. I wasn't quite sure what to expect. I didn't know him at all and hadn't been following what was going happening on The Hill with regards to pathology, although there certainly were issues that applied to medicine as a whole that I was very much aware of.

It turned out his Chief of Staff was the son of a good friend of mine, and as time went on I was meeting with him on a regular basis, at least yearly. I became involved in some fundraising for him and saw him locally as well. Ultimately I did bring him on a laboratory tour in the district. Very soon after his election I was redistricted into his district, so he was indeed my representative after all.

He subsequently ran for the Senate and called me at home to ask me to serve on his finance committee. As you might guess that involved making a lot of phone calls and sending letters. But it was really very exciting, and he won his Senate seat. So I then had to go back to ground zero with my new representative in my district and have actually developed a nice relationship with her.

There are issues that we have been fighting for and it seems as if were fighting for the same old thing, time after time. But when I look back to where we were when I started this process, we've come a long way and we've made progress. It takes persistence and time, but it does work.

The College (Of American Pathologists) is very sensitive to our needs as professionals, our need for time to do other things and to practice our profession. So alerts from the College come infrequently. When they do, it only takes a minute to make a phone call or to put a letter together that you can fax to the legislator's office. In some instances it may take a little more time if you're trying to mobilize the troops by calling some of your colleagues. But for the most part, this is not a large component of my day.

It's Fun

One of the most exciting instances has been meeting and talking with the President of the United States at a Round Table that was held in my community. This was very much a surprise. I got a call from someone who had some Washington connections to ask me about some medical liability issues.

At the time I was serving not only as a member of the College's federal and state affairs committee, but I was also serving as chief of staff at my hospital. This person who was formally a physician but was doing some legislative consulting work, asked me some things and asked if I would be willing to tell some people from Washington what I had just told him.

I said, "Well, when?" and that I would have to check my schedule and he said, "Well it will be next Thursday, and your audience will be the President of the United States." So I promptly said that I thought I could fit it in, and it was quite something. It was my fifteen minutes of fame, I guess. It was really quite exciting to meet with the President and discuss some of the issues that we had concerns about.

Another fun and exciting experience I had was to appear on a morning talk show that is no longer being shown. It was the birthday of George Papanicolaou, who developed the Pap Test. It was just a couple of minutes in which I told the interviewer about the importance of the Pap Test, what a life saving test it was, and it was kind of fun and a little bit silly.

Role Of Money

Money helps to buy you access. At the end of the day, when the Congressman comes back from The Hill and there's a stack of phone messages and a stack of emails, if my name is in that stack and I've been a gracious and loyal contributor, then the odds are pretty good I may get the call back rather than someone that the Congress person has never heard from.

The reality is that to run a campaign takes a lot of money. It's getting into the millions now, and I don't know a way to fix that. There probably are better ways to run campaigns, but currently it takes a lot of money to run a campaign. If you have a relationship with a legislator, it behooves you to make contributions to help that person stay elected and be able to help you.

There are limits to how much we can give and I think most of us are very relieved that there are such limits. The current limit is about $2,300 per election.

To get their attention takes in the range of $250. Certainly $500 or $1,000 is even better. If, like me, you have become linked with your political action committee of your professional organization you can present checks to the legislator from that political action committee and get a little bit more bang for your buck.

Show Me The Money

In the last election I can think of, I had a check from the College's PAC and I got together three or four other local pathologists. We practice in a couple of different hospitals, so it was a nice mix of folks who were politically active or at least interested in becoming active.

We called and made an appointment, told him that we had a check to give him and we would like to meet with him. We met with him in the campaign office. He had doughnuts for us. We spoke briefly about some of our concerns. He spoke about how the campaign was going, and we had doughnuts and coffee and took some pictures and went our way. It was informal.

There had been other instances where I have gone to a large fundraising event, a cocktail party. My Senator has an annual birthday party that is given by his female supporters, including his wife. In some instances I have brought a check from the PAC, and as part of checking in and getting my name tag have presented it to the campaign staff. That's a little less personal, but certainly you get a chance to say hello to the legislator while you're there.

(Author's note: I recommend you find a way to put the check in the politician's hand, so he or she can connect the check with your face. The staff may deposit it without saying a word.)

Get Out Of The Office

Some pathologists get accused of wanting to stay behind our microscopes, but I really enjoy meeting new people with new ideas. Being in politics, I have had the opportunity to meet a lot of people in my community that I might not have interacted with. The medical community at times gets to be a little bit cloistered. But I've met people in all sorts of activities, both in my community and when I come to Washington. I have developed relationships with our Washington office staff.

We need to stop being what one legislator called "invisible doctors." Particularly in my specialty of pathology, a lot of patients and a lot of legislators never know who we are and what we do. I think it would be worthwhile, even if you're not coming to Washington, to contact your legislator about visiting your laboratory.

If your legislator is visiting your hospital on some other task, introduce yourself and offer to show them the laboratory. As events come up in the district it's very easy to get on mailing lists for your legislator, to go to fundraisers, to go to events where he or she is speaking. It's also pretty easy just to call up and make an appointment to see the legislator.

Who Pays Your Salary

You need to remember who's paying your salary. Our patient mix is in large part Medicare and Medicaid. That pay check is very much connected to what happens on Capitol Hill. If you're not a player in what's going on in the Hill and are not aware of legislation that may affect your pocketbook and your ability to provide excellent patient care, then somebody else is going to make these decisions for you. You can play the game or let somebody else make the decisions and deal with the consequences.

Do They Listen To Physicians?

They are very eager to learn. Many legislators find medicine to be a fascinating field. They do not have the basic knowledge about what physicians do every day and how we make decisions. They are gracious and eager to learn, because they have a lot of things on their plate: transportations issues, taxation, insurance issues.

Some of the issues we have, if they're presented rationally in a non-emotional fashion and are linked to the health of the voters back in their district, can really have an impact.

Demeanor Of Physicians

If we try to make ourselves educators, if we try to teach, if we try to enlighten legislators about what we do and why we do it, perhaps this power play will not become an issue. Even with our patients, there are times when physicians become too patronizing and need to create more of a partnership with their patients.

If we view our work and our interaction with legislators as a partnership, as a learning experience, we can make it work. After all, we have things to learn too about how the political process works and why some things happen on The Hill and some don't and why things take so long.

Physicians' Income Colors The Discussion

We do make a good living, and that's part of why I give back to my profession by doing things like this. But I'm working harder today than I was four or five years ago, and I'm making less. I'm living comfortably, but I still have overhead in my practice. I still have bills to pay, and those bills are coming and are not being lowered just because my income is less.

What is happening in some practices is that physicians are having to limit the number of patients they see from the Medicare and/or Medicaid population. In some instances doctors actually lose money on each Medicaid patient they see for certain procedures and certain tests. This ultimately will limit access to medical care for some of our most needy patients. If the neediest of our population does not have access to medical care then we're really going to be in a fix.

Carol Dittman, M.D.

Dr. Carol Dittman is a pathologist I met when she was in Washington, DC lobbying for the American College of Pathologists. This is the story she told right after her first ever visit to Capitol Hill.

Up The Hill

The College of American Pathologists contacted me through a CAP Action Alert, which was an e-mail. I mailed a letter in response to that Action Alert to Rep. Joe Bonner, asking him to co-sponsor the bill, HR1237, which concerned cytology proficiency testing.

He responded with a letter saying he would consider co-sponsoring. I scheduled a meeting with him here in Washington. When I entered his office he informed me he had already co-sponsored the bill based on the letter that I had written him.

I also met with Senator Shelby's staff and Senator Shelby came into the room and we had a great discussion. I also met with the staff for Senator Jeff Sessions.

Once we had decided Rep. Bonner was on the same page with the cytology proficiency bill, we discussed him coming to my laboratory and allowing me to show him how these Pap smears are processed. He is very ready and willing to do that in the next few weeks since this is a current topic. So he is going to come do a laboratory tour with us.

It was much easier than I had anticipated, and I believe I can do this and look forward to the next time. They were very receptive and engaging. It was an exciting time.

Update:

I contacted Dr. Dittman some time after this interview and she had some interesting updates. Rep. Bonner did come visit her lab and spent about a half day there talking with employees and learning about Pap smears among other things. He had lunch with hospital administrators and other employees. In 2008, Dr. Dittman moved to a new job in Oklahoma. When I talked with her, she was about to meet with members of Congress from there.

Ben Regalado, Practice Manager

Ben Regalado worked in Maryland for Hospital Corporation of America as regional administrator for physician services. I met him at a seminar on politics for the anesthesia section of Medical Group Management Association.

Getting Started

In my high school government class, I had a very demanding teacher. He was one of those they tell you about: You don't want Mr. Cochran. I got Mr. Cochran. But he made it really interesting and exciting. Mr. Cochran said we're going to take a tour of City Hall.

I went up to him and said, "Mr. Cochran, since we're going to City Hall and there is this big debate going on about transportation and rail, why don't we get one of the city council members to come talk to us?"

He looked me in the eye and said, "Mr. Regalado, that is a fine idea. Why don't you set it up."

So I did. And I realized even as a teenager that this was fun and I enjoyed it.

Then I had a chance to do an internship on a gubernatorial campaign. That was my first brush with glory. The political strategist that beat us was a young whippersnapper named Karl Rove.

Politicians Are Real People

I had a friend who was really passionate about some issues and she wanted to run for County Commissioner. I said, "Well, I worked on a campaign one time. I can drive you around and help you put up yard signs." Before I knew what had happened I was managing her campaign. I realized, this is still fun. I got to meet a lot of new people, to meet the staff of members of Congress and talk with members of Congress.

These politicians are real life people. They are not the television caricatures. They're firefighters. Some of them are teachers. A lot of them are lawyers. You have a relationship every day with patients. You can have that relationship with politicians.

Sure, there are some bad apples out there, but most people in politics want to do a good job and want to be of service. Sure, you've got to have a big ego to run for office. But one-to-one they are very personable. They want to do what is best for their constituents.

Washington Staff

In Washington you deal a lot with young staff. I tell people to be prepared. This country is run by a bunch of 26-year-olds. They are very passionate, very dedicated to the political system. They are not getting paid a lot of money. They work tremendous hours trying to do good things for their country.

That lowly staff person you talk with today will be chief of staff for a very important committee chair you want to see in the future. The lady who answers the phone in (Maryland) Sen. Barbara Mikulski's office is the mother of the governor.

Making a Difference

When I was in North Carolina we got the managers together and got a bill passed. We got a win. You can do this. Now I'm in Maryland and it's the same thing.

The percent of anesthesiologists communicating at all with politicians is probably 10% or less. I hope all those are effective, but it's probably less.

Get Out Of The Box

Anesthesiologists need to get out of the OR. The type medicine they deliver is very important to patients, but it's episodic. You don't have that relationship building process that goes on when you meet with your patients again and again. Sometimes they apply that process to political relationships and they are not building relationships over time.

They see it as episodic: Medicare, tort reform. They tackle it issue by issue. They need to move beyond the episodic approach to a long-term approach. That's hard when you've had 12 years training in an episodic manner.

Two things need to happen. You need to develop a passion among anesthesiologists. That happens when a peer has a passion and recruits them. The second thing is a passionate practice administrator to support them. The anesthesiologist's job is taking care of patients. They don't have time to organize the letters and follow everything in great detail. A good manager and a passionate doctor can make the difference for a group.

Make Politics Your Job

I put it this way, if politics is not in your job description, let's look at the numbers. Medicare. Medicaid. HMO law. Workers comp. That's your revenue. Then let's look at things like EEOC regulations and how much time residents can work. How can you manage that more effectively? Politics has to be part of your job. It is part of your job because you are either responding to what the politicians are doing or you are at the table helping to shape the decisions that affect your practice.

For those who think they can't do it, think of it this way: Every day in your practice you are dealing with people just like the politicians. You are managing physicians. You know how to herd cats.

What Makes A Difference

I'm there. I'm at the committee meetings. I'm sending the letters. I'm shaking their hand. They get to see me. They realize this is the guy from anesthesia. They see you. And they see you again. And then you're invited to the meetings. You're invited to the table.

Politics doesn't belong to the guy who shows up with a check. A lot of people believe that, but that's not it. It belongs to the guy who shows up.

Show Politicians The Facts

Practice administrators can show the numbers. We are a 15-20 million dollar business in your district. We create jobs: doctors, nurses, medical assistants. We are an important part of this community. We support the hospital. We need to convey that this is not about a doctor's paycheck; it's much deeper than that.□

Melody Mena, Registered Nurse

When I met Melody Mena, I was working for AORN, the Association of peri-Operative Registered Nurses. The organization and the nurses had serious issues with Medicare reimbursement to the point their very existence was threatened. They were being replaced with less-trained and less-well-paid caregivers.

Melody is a perfect example of someone who went from zero political participation to a leader in a national organization. This first segment is from a speech she gave at a Washington fly-in/lobby day. The second segment is from a follow-up interview.

Clueless

I had no clue. I did not know any elected official at all. Not even their names.

I voted. I did. But I didn't know who I was voting for. That was it. That was as close as I got.

So I went onto the web and started looking around and I thought, I wonder who my representative is?

I found out that my representative was Mac Collins.

I thought, well, this is pretty cool.

So I started reading about him and doing some research and I found his phone number and I called his office.

I said, "Hi, this is Melody Mena. I'm the president of my local chapter of the Association of Operating Room nurses. We are going to have this really great big kick-off meeting in your district and we are going to invite doctors and nurses and CEOs of hospitals and they all want to hear Mac Collins talk about healthcare, so we want him to speak to us."

Maybe This Could Work

And they said, "This sounds interesting. We'll get back to you." They called back later and said, "Yeah, he'd like to speak to your group."

I said, "Great, this is wonderful." I hung up the phone and called an emergency meeting of my newly elected association board and told them I had sort of made up this thing that we were supposed to do in five weeks.

They were trying to find a way to write an impeachment process into the bylaws because they realized they had a big thing on their hands.

Well, while I was talking to Mac Collins' office about the arrangements, I had to say we changed the place for the meeting because we are going to have extra people attending that we didn't plan on. 'Course, I never had a place, I had just made it up. They asked where the meeting was and I had to tell them something.

While we were talking, I said, "Can I have an appointment with him, like, two weeks after the meeting?"

They said sure.

So I called AORN and told them I was meeting with my member of Congress and asked them, "What do I say?" I had no clue what to say to this man or what to talk about.

They told me I needed to talk to him about HCFA.

So I went and got some friends of mine and dragged them along. There was no way I was going by myself.

We talked about the operating room nurse and what we do and why it is so important. We told him about the HCFA thing and reimbursement and what it means to patients and health care.

She Gets A Strong Reaction

Mac Collins was absolutely horrified.

He said, "I will write a letter and I will get it to you." He faxed me that letter the next day.

I was dumfounded. So I called him back to thank him for the letter and asked for another appointment. So I got another appointment, and then another, and I would bring somebody different every time.

Then I found his itinerary on the web site. I started showing up at every single town hall meeting, every parade. I would drag my family along and I would be waving and yelling, "Hi Mac!"

He would be on the back of a car going down the road and look at me and think, there she is again.

My husband said, "Melody, he thinks you're stalking him."

So finally I went in to see if he would sponsor AORN's bill, the major legislation we wanted. I was ready to argue with him. I had all my facts together.

I went in and said, "Mac, I want you to introduce this legislation. It's ready. We need to do it. I want you to introduce this legislation."

And he said, "Okay."

Epilogue

We went to the grand finale of his campaign and gave him a T-shirt and a plaque, signed by almost every nurse in his district. We thanked him for everything he'd done for us.

It was the simplest thing in the world.

He was moved to tears because he knew how hard we had worked and how much we cared about him.

We showed him that as nurses we may not have tons of money, but we have lots of spirit and we will be there for him, because he's never turned his back on us.

That's why he is such a champion for us today.

I know that if we can do this with one representative in the House, we can do it with every single one of them.

We just have to let them know we're there. Half of them don't even know we exist.

I realized they put their pants on the same way I do, one leg at time.

Later on, I realized that if I were a senator sitting in my office and somebody came in and said I need you to vote this way on nuclear fusion I would look at them, like, "Okay, I need a little bit more information. I have no idea what you're talking about."

It's Up To Us

It's the same with us. They have no idea what we are talking about. It's up to nurses to fix the problem. The policy makers do not know how to fix it.

I have had a blast. I have met so many interesting people. I realized one day that all my friends were nurses. After I got started in politics I have a friend who is a financial agent, one who is a mortgage broker, one who owns half the county I live in. He rents houses. I have a friend who is an airplane mechanic.

It's so interesting to meet new kinds of people. I went to this big function and Mac Collins introduced me to the Speaker of the House. I noticed there were these two guys there with these little coiled wires in their ear. It was amazing.

I had never in my life seen secret service people before except in the movies.

It's like a breath of fresh air to meet people from different walks of life who care about things and who are there to make a difference in the way our country and our local government is run.

Every politician I have met can relate to me in some way and I can relate to them. We see them in the media and they become some kind of figurehead that's very intimidating. But when you meet them, they are normal people.

Most of the general public doesn't get involved in politics and doesn't like it. They think all politicians are crooks. That's not true. I've been surprised and found quite the contrary. They will at least listen to you.

There are big differences between Republicans and Democrats, but they all have the people in mind, just in different ways.

The Academics: What Scientific Research Shows about Grassroots

Michael Lord, PhD.

Michael Lord, PhD, was Director of Flow Institute for International Studies, and Associate Professor of Management for Babcock Graduate School of Management, Wake Forest University. He conducted a study to find out what influences politicians.

We talked with directors of corporations, administrative assistants, lobbyists for associations and corporations. We promised anonymity and confidentiality to get as much input and as honest opinion as possible.

We worked hard to remove any bias from the process. So one of the things that we did was interview and survey a number of former legislative assistants and former legislative directors who no longer worked on Capitol Hill. That way, they wouldn't have to worry about how their opinions would reflect on themselves or their congressional offices.

What we found was consistent across the board from all the different groups, from lobbyists, from corporate public affairs executives and from legislative directors and administrative assistants. Grass roots plays an incredibly important role in the public policy process in terms of influencing legislative decision-making. It is the single most influential tactic in influencing the decision-making.

Grassroots is the education and mobilization of different groups of stakeholders to contact their legislators to voice their opinion and influence public policy. For a company it can be anything from employees to shareholders to salespeople to distributors to anyone who has a stake in an issue. If they can be educated and then motivated and mobilized to contact their legislators and make their voice heard, that is what grass roots is all about.

E-mail Least Effective

E-mail is usually at the bottom of the list in terms of effectiveness. Precisely because it is so easy. The cheaper, simpler, easier it is in terms of a means of communicating with Congress, the less likely it is to have impact. That's because it doesn't demonstrate much effort, much caring about the issue. So a form e-mail is going to have very limited impact.

On the other hand, a sincere well-written e-mail in the words of the actual constituent is going to have an impact. But it doesn't communicate the context and the sincerity of the feeling as well as something like a hand typed or handwritten letter.

(Author's note: See earlier comments advising against postal mail to Congress.)

Legislators and their staff want to know the strength of the feeling of the constituent. They also want to know how informed the constituent is on the issue, because that tells them how important it is for them.

Power Of One Voice

They also want to know what is the impact in the district or state on the constituent. Is the person's job at stake? That is probably the most significant factor that legislator or staff will consider in how to vote on an issue.

If they hear from a constituent whose job is threatened by an issue before Congress, that has an enormous impact. That would be one good example of understanding why a constituent feels the way they do. The more important it is for the constituent and the more they make that clear to the legislator, then the more impact it is going to have. The competition varies. It ebbs and flows depending on what issues are before Congress and what is going on in Congress. In general, most offices don't hear from very many constituents on public policy or specific issues. It is in the low single digits percentage wise of constituents who contact their legislators for any public policy related reason.

So this idea that one voice can't be heard or that a group of a dozen voices can't be heard is just not true. In fact, 10 or 12 well placed contacts at the appropriate point of the public policy process can have enormous impact. The cynicism in the US today results in fewer and fewer people participating, so the ones who do voice their feedback have more impact than ever.

In terms of the technical and economic details, the professional lobbyists and corporate executive, people of that sort, will provide a lot of front-end input to the legislation. Then at the end of the process, when it actually comes up for a vote, whether it is a committee vote or at the end of the process in terms of being voted out of the House or the Senate, grassroots play an absolutely critical role in determining how each individual Congress person or senator is going to vote.

Some Tactics Can Backfire

It is a little bit different with the committee chairman. If you are not a direct constituent of theirs, chances are you are not going to be heard directly. The best way may be to go through your senator or representative and try to use their influence on the committee chair.

If your senator or representative is on the committee, or even if they are not on the committee, they still have influence. They call it 'log rolling', trading favors and 'you scratch my back, and I'll scratch yours.' So the best way to influence a specific committee may be to contact your senator or your representative and have them carry your voice to that chairperson. Those constituents can have an incredible amount of influence. But there is reason for caution in trying to influence those committee chairmen from outside the district.

If you tried to manufacture grassroots feedback that is not really sincere just because you are trying to influence the house speaker or the committee chairs, it can backfire and have a negative impact. The committee chairs have less time and less attention than any other member of Congress, because they are so busy. So only sincere and authentic feedback from real constituents is going to have much impact.

If you live in the district or the state of the committee chair, you do have a special influence over public policy, even more so than just your average constituent. They (committee chairs) have a much louder voice in Congress and you have a much larger voice in trying to influence what they hear and what they consider to be important. If you are a constituent of a committee chair, you have a lot more opportunity to have much more impact than your average constituent.

Money Talks, But Quietly

People assume money makes the world go around in politics. It is an important influence, but it is more in the background. It is something that has always been there, probably always be there, no matter how many laws or campaign finance reforms are passed, so it does play an important role, but it is more part of the infrastructure of politics.

Everyone's got money, everyone gives money, everyone needs money to run their campaign. But when you have Bell on one side of an issue giving $5,000 to a campaign and you have AT&T on the other side of the issue giving $5,000 for the campaign, who wins in that situation?

In that case Bell might win because they have a lot more employees in that Congressperson's district or state and they have those employees and those managers, maybe even the shareholders, contact their legislator. So with money you have kind of an arms race that no one really wins.

It does not have nearly the influence that people think that it does, and in part that is because of this arms race mentality where everyone is getting money and almost everybody is giving, so no one wins.

Surprised About Role Of Money

I went in with the expectation that money played a much more important role than it actually does. The political science research is based on campaign contributions. It is easy to get that data. The Federal Election Commission gives you computer tapes with all the data on how much Congressman X got and from whom, so it is very easy to run statistics. It is also easy for the media to get a hold of those figures and splash them on the front page.

Most of what you see in the media and in the political science literature is about money and about how much influence money has on the political process. But what they miss is everything that is going on in the background that isn't quite so glamorous or scandalous as the money changing hands.

I went into this research with the assumption that money plays much more of a role in politics than I actually found. I was surprised, but also I wasn't surprised because of my experience with grassroots politics. The research brought me back to where I started.

One of the things we taught in campaign management and our schools on how to win political campaigns was that money does not win campaigns. Votes win election campaigns. You can spend a lot of money and not get very many votes.

A lot of people don't understand that money and the policy process are separated. They are legally divided. Bribery is not legal. There is a distinct separation between a legislative campaign organization that takes political contributions and the office on

Capitol Hill, which actually makes public policy and makes legislation. Most offices have a firewall and it is sincere and real in most cases. You read about the exceptions where there is a scandal or where there is some implicit bribery.

There are two distinct parts of a Congressman and what they do. One is the campaign organization. The other is their office on Capitol Hill that makes public policy. There is a firewall between those two offices. In most cases one doesn't know much of what the other is doing, and part of that is for legal reasons. It is also for ethical reasons. Bribery is neither legal nor ethical in the US Congress, despite all the headlines.

You Read About The Exceptions

What you read about are the exceptions where the money gets mingled with public policy decisions. But in most cases, and certainly in all activity that is legal, giving money to a campaign organization is not necessarily going to have much impact or even be known about by those who are influencing policy.

They tend to know where the money is coming from in congressional offices when there is a donation to their campaign organization, but that is usually because it's their constituent and it's an important constituent for the legislator. So they already know that constituent. And they are probably giving because they are an important constituent with an interest in the legislator, and they are already having an influence.

Maybe they are grateful for the influence they are having, so they will give the campaign contributions. The problem is that people confuse it and see it the other way around, that someone has given the campaign a contribution and then they have influence.

One comment that came up frequently in surveying and interviewing staffers on Capitol Hill was, in their own words, "Spare me stupid reminders of past financial support." So when you are wanting to influence legislation and wanting your opinion to be heard, the staff really don't care about, and in fact resent it, when you mention that you gave a campaign contribution and you mention how frequently and how much and how many times.

The staffers on the Hill feel they don't deal with campaign organization matters and fundraising. So that was a very common comment: do not try to influence me or influence our decision by repeatedly and forcefully reminding me of your campaign contributions.

Creating Impact

Powerful communication from constituents usually involves a very personal, strongly felt message. For example, when someone's job is at stake, or when it involves medical research and someone's son or daughter has a particular disease, something of that sort. Those are the most influential for emotional reasons as well as for electoral reasons.

You want to demonstrate that you have a very sincere heartfelt interest with your story. You also want to make it obvious that the legislator is doing the right thing – and maybe look like a hero or champion for a particular cause, whether it is jobs in the district or medical research funding, whatever the case may be.

Another thing that can be really effective is home district or home state plant visits or company visits. News stations are likely to cover it. You combine a lot of backslapping and handshaking at the plant with people who may be voters. They are also employees of the company. In general you make a good story and you make good PR for the legislator.

Talking With Staff

It is another misperception that you have a right or you need to talk to the legislator directly. They only have so much time. There are a lot of people competing for their time and attention, and you can have just as much impact if not more so by talking to the right staff members at the right time.

It is not the case that your voice is not heard unless you talk to the legislator directly. Talking to key staff members can be just as effective, even more effective. They are more likely to remember and take notes on what you are saying, maybe even more so than the legislator themselves.

When a congressional office hears from someone, if it is not a constituent it has practically zero impact. There are a few exceptions, for example, if someone is an expert on an issue. If they are a top scientist in the country or something of an expert on a technical issue.

Contact from a constituent is taken very seriously, and congressional offices quickly sort out which contact has come from constituents. The first mechanism they use to screen and judge feedback is, "Is this from a constituent?" So that is the first thing they are going to look at and consider. If it is from a constituent it will get read; it will get heard. If it is not from a constituent it is not worth much.

If you are not a constituent you might have an important issue and a good message, but everyone has limited time and attention and everyone has their own self-interest. It is not the best use of that legislator's time and attention and of their staff's time and attention, and it is not in their self-interest to pay attention to feedback from a non-constituent. So they spend their time and effort responding to constituents.

What Works And What Doesn't

The most effective approach would be to go visit that office in Washington DC or go and visit that office in the home district or the home state.

Given that most people aren't going to be able to do that, letters are still incredibly effective. Just a plain old hand-written or typed letter, especially if they are not form letters. They are the most effective.

(Author's note: Remember, don't use postal mail to communicate with Congress.)

Phone calls are very effective as well. Then you start getting into the media that are less effective, blast faxes and then things like e-mails, and then mass mail devices, postcards and pre-printed letters where you tick the boxes and that sort.

When you want to think about how to be most effective, whatever type of communication mechanism shows the most sincerity, the most effort, the most thought and the most care in terms of the message you are trying to communicate, is going to have the most impact. The type of media you use signifies how intensely you feel about an issue, how informed you are about an issue and how likely you are to follow up on that issue.

If you visit in person, that signifies that you are very interested in the issue, you are very informed about it and you are very likely to follow up on it. If you just send a form e-mail or if you return a mass printed postcard, it doesn't show very much interest or very much effort and you are not very likely to follow up on it, whether the legislator votes your way or not.

Professional lobbyists and executives who lobby play a very important role in providing information, primarily detailed economics and technical information. They are appreciated by the legislators and staff, but it doesn't tell you which way they should vote. It just gives them the technical and economic details. When they really want to know how they should vote on the issue that is where grassroots comes in and plays a really important role.

Companies that have a large presence in any legislator's home district or state have a lot of influence and it is mostly through their employment base, through the people that they directly employ, through suppliers, things of that sort. So companies who employ in a legislator's home district state can have a lot of influence.

Volume Of Communications Makes A Difference

The amount of feedback a legislator receives plays an important role, but it is not just a matter of weighing how many letters or postcards they got. The quality matters just as much if not more than the quantity. So the goal of grassroots is not to see how many responses we can get sent back, but it is to have sheer quality grassroots feedback. One well-written, informed, individual letter could be worth 100 postcards.

Within the 2-3% of constituents who actually contact their congressional office in any given year, probably less than 1% are about any specific economic or business related legislation. Much of it is about individual casework, matters like Social Security or a hot button social issue like abortion. The ones who contact Congress, who engage in grassroots, become incredibly important because they symbolize that there is or there may be a larger group of people out there who feel the same way on an issue. But even if they aren't representative, if that big silent majority feels differently on an issue, it doesn't necessarily matter much to a legislator.

That's because they ARE silent; they don't care about an issue, they are not informed about it, they don't even know how they feel about it. So even if the grassroots contact is a minority in some sense, if you were to poll the whole constituent base, that minority is still incredibly important because those other people don't know or don't care.

The squeaky wheel gets the grease. The member of Congress can't know how those other people feel or whether they care because they never hear from them.

What Makes A Difference?

To make an issue a priority item for a congressional office, the number of contacts needed varies dramatically from office to office. But in many cases just a few contacts maybe 5, 10 or 12 contacts at the right time can have a critical influence on a congressional office.

For example, when an issue is just getting started or when a congressional office is not even aware of a particular issue, 5, 10 or 12 sincerely written letters or sincere well-spoken phone calls can have a tremendous impact.

There is definitely a grassroots arms race as more companies, associations and public interest groups have realized that grassroots is very effective. So everyone tries to mount a grassroots effort.

That is another key reason why Congress is deluged with so many communications these days, so it is all relative. If 100 letters had an impact 10 years ago, it may take 1,000 today, but it is all relative in terms of everyone drowning each other out. There are too many voices, a lot of noise.

So it comes down to quality often rather than quantity. Quality letters, quality phone calls, quality communications of any kind will always get attention and will always have influence.

Relationships Matter

Ongoing grassroots programs are important to build a relationship. If you tried to respond on a particular issue and a staff member or legislator has never heard from you before and doesn't know who you are, who your company is or who your association is, the chances are that your letters and phone calls are not going to get the attention they deserve.

If you have an ongoing grassroots program to communicate with legislator offices, they will know you. Your letters and phone calls will get through the clutter; they will be heard. So that is the difference between doing ad-hoc grassroots programs at the last minute, which is more typical of what most associations and organizations do, than having a sincere ongoing grassroots program.

If you could deliver 100 sincere letters from constituents, you would have a major impact on that office and on their priorities.

Corporate Executives

Corporate Executives play at least two key roles in grass roots. First, they have a tremendous amount of prestige. They are high profile, so they are likely to get access to a congressional office and probably to the legislator themselves. They can plant the seed or lay the groundwork for telling a legislator what is the key issue.

The second key role they play is that grassroots programs that are most effective are those in which top executives are supportive and in which they play an active role. It means they know and understand the importance of the grassroots. They value it. They make it part of the strategy of the company to influence public policy through grass roots.

Influence Of Media

The local media play a really important role in influencing legislators in their decisions. But you need to use it as part of a larger program. You need to have a media relationship program, things like doing editorial board meetings, op-ed pieces, letters to the editor, as well as a grassroots program.

Most legislators and their staff don't know exactly how their constituents feel. They can take a poll, which gives some sort of shallow indication of how people feel, but they don't really know what is important to the constituents and how important it is. That is why grassroots is so important, because on most issues, most legislators and their staff simply don't know how their constituents feel.

(Author's note: Politicians are rightly skeptical of polls, even when they use them. Or they may be skeptical, rightly, of their constituents. One well-respected poll, the National Science Foundation's "Science and Engineering Indicators 2006," found that 29 percent of respondents said the Sun goes around the Earth.)

Polls are very limited. Some offices conduct polling of their district to see what people feel and what is important to them. If you ask someone how they feel about a particular issue they will respond. They will check a box, but it doesn't mean they really care about that issue, that they even know what the issue is. That is where grassroots is different; it is richer and much more meaningful than a poll.

It also indicates whether or not that person is likely to participate in politics. Someone replying to a poll is not likely to be politically active; they are just doing so because someone shoved a clipboard in their face.

But someone who bothers to write a personal letter to Congress or spend 15 minutes on the phone talking to staff, they are by definition "politically active." That group of people who are politically active are also the ones who are going to be voting on Election Day or working for a campaign or against a campaign when the next election comes around.

Be One of the Few, the Effective

Less than 2-3% of constituents will actually write a letter or make a phone call in any given year.

E-mail is great because it is fast, cheap and easy. But it also is one of the less effective means of communicating with Congress, precisely because it is so fast, cheap and easy. So e-mail in general has not been very effective so far, but that is changing. E-mail is becoming more effective as people learn how to use it better, and as more congressional offices learn how to incorporate responding to e-mail in their systems.

The volume of communication in the congressional offices is definitely on the increase, largely due to e-mail. But when Congress gets deluged with millions of e-mails as they have been, those millions as a group do not get much attention and don't have much influence. They get devalued if not discarded. Spamming a congressional office or all congressional offices with e-mail is not effective, and in fact can backfire and have a negative impact.

Other Academic Views

Bruce C. Wolpe and Bertram J. Levine

Bruce C. Wolpe and Bertram J. Levine wrote a great book for Congressional Quarterly (CQ Press) called "Lobbying Congress: How The System Works." I recommend you buy it.

From the second edition:

Lobbying does not come naturally to most business people, whether corporate CEOs or entrepreneurs. They are used to being "somebody" within their communities.... They are used to having some degree of control over their professional lives and to being important within their most proximate spheres of business activity – their own companies.

For such people Capitol Hill can be a demoralizing and ego-shattering place. They find themselves sitting in dingy anterooms, one of several pleaders, waiting to see a congressional staff person not yet five years out of college... Instead of being "somebody," they feel like "nobody"...

The more effort a person puts into a communication with a member of Congress, the more impact that communication is likely to have when it reaches The Hill... The message of concern works on a legislator at two levels. First, because the legislator may see added legitimacy in the issue, he or she may decide to take a more aggressive role in supporting, opposing or modifying relevant legislation; thus a useful ally would be recruited for the legislative cause. Second, the member has every reason to assume that a correlation exists between the amount of effort one is willing to put into a personal communication and how likely that person is to remember the legislator's response at election time...

(Congressional offices) have become increasingly aggressive in defending themselves... many offices now spot check communications by calling people whose names and addresses appear on letters or were given during the course of phone conversations. The first objective is to verify authenticity; the second is to gain an understanding of how much the constituent really knows and cares about the issue. One office reported, "It's amazing how many callers say things like 'I don't really know much about it. The boss just asked that we make the call. He even let us use his office phone.'" Such gratuitous information obviously undermines the credibility of the campaign.

Antoinette J. Pole

Antoinette J. Pole surveyed hundreds of legislators in Vermont and New York for her doctoral dissertation at City University of New York titled E-mocracy: Information Technology & State Legislatures.

Excerpted with her permission:

The importance of maintaining and facilitating face-to-face contact for lobbying remains paramount, not to be replaced by information technologies.

Interest group respondents in both states overwhelmingly rejected the notion that e-mail allows their organization to exert more pressure or influence over state legislators, leadership and committee chairs... 50% of interest group respondents in Vermont and 66% in New York reported that the Internet is the least effective method of lobbying.

In an apologetic manner a state legislator in New York told me that while he tries to get to e-mail sometimes as many five days would pass without checking his account. This is largely because of how much time it takes to filter e-mail; meaning deleting non-constituent e-mail and advertisements and scanning messages for viruses.

In New York, staff told me that there is a perception that a reply sent by e-mail is "less official" than a reply sent via US Post, which appears on letterhead and contains the state legislator's signature.

These findings do not support the hypothesis that interest groups can exert influence through e-mail and the Internet.

The Lobbyists: Paid Professionals Who Usually Don't Smoke Cigars

Lobbyists come to the process both passionately and dispassionately. They all have deep, powerful beliefs about what they do. Many are personally committed to the cause they represent. In many ways they are like lawyers (many are lawyers, but by no means all). They are hired to defend a client and they succeed on their ability to make the best possible case for that client, regardless of guilt or innocence.

A term lobbyists use to describe themselves time and again is "hired gun." Politicians and staff view them that way too. They often like lobbyists, have close relationships with them, respect them and trust them. But everyone knows the lobbyist may also be working for the other side a day later, just as a lawyer may work as a prosecutor and then switch to defending criminals.

Their message to politicians is always weaker than that of a true believer, a stakeholder, a participant, a constituent. It's like the defense lawyer who does not say to a judge, "My client is innocent" but rather, "Our position is that he is innocent" or "My client maintains he has done nothing wrong." Huge numbers of lobbyists ply their trade in Washington competing for time with 535 elected officials and their staff.

How Many Lobbyists?

Just how many is not clear. CNN reported that there are "more than 37,000 registered lobbyists." The Christian Science Monitor cited "39,402." The Seattle Times has "32,890." USA Today, "more than 32,000." Sen. Carl Levin (D-MI) referred to "more than 30,000." The Senate Office of Public Records (SOPR), the agency responsible for receiving lobbyist registrations and publishing them online, reports 32,890 registered lobbyists last time I checked.

Debra Mayberry, president of Columbia Books Inc., publisher of several directories listing professionals, including lobbyists and association executives, puts the number at about 11,500. The difference is, her company only counts unduplicated, active lobbyists. Having used her directories for years, I think she's probably more on the mark than other estimates. The actual number in Washington and your state doesn't matter. What's important is that there are so many the competition for the time and attention of elected officials is intense.

How do people become lobbyists? Usually by accident. There is almost no formal training for the job and no high school counselor will ever say, "You should be a lobbyist."

Someone who has solid experience on a House or Senate committee might be able to leave government and take a lobbying job that starts at $300,000 a year.

To retain one of the big lobbying firms might cost an association or corporation $15,000 to $30,000 a month or more, depending on the activity.

But there is a limit to what lobbyists can do no matter how many people and how much money they represent and how good the relationship with a politician is. A politician's most important loyalty and dependence is on the voters back home. No politician ever got defeated for making a lobbyist angry, but plenty have been sent packing for making voters angry. That's why your role as a volunteer advocate is so important.

Dustin Corcoran

I spoke with Dustin Corcoran, Vice President of Government Relations, California Medical Association, at his office in Sacramento. He gives a good perspective on the role of a lobbyist.

There are five lobbyists here at CMA in addition to myself, and a couple of contract lobbyists. It's not that legislators don't hear from us. They hear from us just about every day. But what's important is hearing directly from physicians, the person in the district who actually has to deal with the issues and the consequences of legislation passed here in Sacramento.

They know that I'm paid to advocate on behalf of physicians and so to be able to hear from constituents directly is vitally important. In fact, it carries more weight, because they know that somebody's taking time out of their very busy day to contact them and express an opinion on legislation.

If a legislator has heard from physicians before I walk into the office it makes a tremendous difference. If a number of constituents have called about legislation, when I walk in they are eager to hear and listen to me. What it means is I'm finding a way to give a good answer to their constituents.

Say they've gotten 10 phone calls from physicians in their district. That's critical because when I walk in, I'm telling them here's how you're going to be able to give a good answer to the physicians in your district. They are very eager to write a letter back and say that they delivered on behalf of their constituents. So it makes the reception much more welcoming when we walk in and it's not the first time they've heard about the issue. They know it's an issue that's important to their constituents back in the district.

Politicians Want To Hear from You

What they want to hear from a practicing physician in their district is the effect legislation is going to have on their ability to be able to practice medicine. That's the key difference.

As professional lobbyists we are able to wade through the minutia of legislation and talk about what's on page 7 of the bill, but what they're looking for from constituents is an understanding of how it's going to impact patients and the ability to deliver quality care in their district. Just a few bullet points is often enough to communicate to the legislator effectively. Very often they will hear from a constituent and then call and ask us for more information and more detail on what their constituent called about.

It makes our job easier here in Sacramento when they know they're going to vote with physicians or against physicians; they have to go back and explain that vote to somebody that they've met or somebody that they've seen face to face.

That's not to say that phone calls and letters aren't effective. But even more effective is developing a personal relationship with the legislators so they know that they're going to see you at the next community event or in some other context back in the district and have to look somebody in the face, somebody that they have a relationship with, and explain why they did what they did. It's much more comfortable for a legislator to be able to go back to that next community breakfast and tell a physician, "I took care of you on that bill" or, "I was able to deliver for you on that. I know that was a critical issue for you."

Politicians Want To Make People Happy

Legislators always want to be able to deliver good news as opposed to bad news. When we're battling insurance companies and some of the other folks that we often do battle with here in Sacramento, it's very difficult for the insurance companies to be able to put a human face on the issue. They don't have a sympathetic face back in the district that's going to be seen at the next event. Physicians, when they do engage and get active, provide that human face that legislators are going to have to see and interact with.

The fact that physicians often have a very good income makes some issues difficult. It's probably one of the biggest difficulties physicians have in advocating, because it's true; they are wealthy, particularly compared to what most legislators make and what their constituents make.

Physicians are expected to make money. It's widely perceived that's it's okay and we want them to make money. □But at the same time, to simply discuss pocketbook issues isn't always a winning strategy.

A better way to handle it is to talk about the effect it's going to have on access to care and what it means for patients in the district. Are they going to be able to see a physician? Are they going to be able to see the best physician? Or are we going to create a two-tier system where those folks who may be on the lower end of the income spectrum are forced to seek care in an emergency department or some other venue that may not be the best?

The way to handle that is refocus the issue on access to care and what it means for patients ability to see a quality physician without having to directly discuss pocketbook issues.

Individual Stories Make The Difference

Our President Elect was having a difficult time being re-enrolled as a Medi-Cal provider because he had moved offices – within the same office suite. He had been a Medi-Cal provider in good standing for a long time. But he had to go through a very laborious process to be able to continue to provide Medi-Cal to patients, even though providers provide that service at a loss in this state.

So we got him up here to testify in front of legislators and to personalize that story about what it means for physicians to go through this incredible bureaucracy to do the right thing in providing care to an underserved community. It showed how the state makes it even more difficult to provide care on top of the appallingly low reimbursement that the state pays.

That awakened legislators to a problem they otherwise would have known nothing about. It was a backwater bureaucratic issue from a legislative point of view, yet that personalization of the story really brought it to the forefront in the legislator's minds and caused them to pass legislation to address that issue.

What you need to do is to think about what's going to impact the legislator, what's going to stick in their mind. If you can do something that personalizes the issue, crystallizes it, that shows what it means to not just you, but to the population at large and to the district, that has a massive impact.

Because everything else might be equal, we might be able to counter the opposition in terms of how many lobbyists that they put up and how many resources they put up, to try and influence legislation here in Sacramento. But the key is if we can turn out physicians and have physicians provide those stories.

That always puts us over the top. It's always a struggle to find physicians because they're very busy and have lives that are very much outside of the political spectrum. They need to remember how important legislation is to their ability to be able to continue to practice good medicine in the state.

Failure to engage causes bad outcomes, and we're always here as staff, for CMA, fighting that. But when physicians engage we win. It's always a big help to have those personal stories from the district. Legislators do respond, they do pay attention, and they pay attention a lot more to us as professional staff when individual physicians are participating at the district level.

Site Visits Are High Impact

One of the best things to do is to give a tour of your offices to a legislator. Most legislators don't have a background in medicine and don't have a lot of familiarity with the medical process. So being able to walk through an emergency room, to walk through a pediatric office or an oncologist's office or any specialty is fascinating. It provides you an opportunity in a short period of time to bond with the legislator.

You'll be amazed that many legislators, after having done that, will call you directly to seek your advice and input on issues affecting medicine. Now you've now developed a direct line to that legislator.

That's probably one of the most effective things you can do, because then they not only understand you as an individual, but they understand the challenges facing your practice and have seen the place where you practice.

Short of that it may be as easy as taking them to breakfast, or to coffee, or showing up at one of their events. It's always a good way to establish a rapport with a legislator. They're always looking for informed constituents to be able to bounce ideas off. Taking a little time out of your day and visiting with them means a lot.

Money Talk

Money and politics are inseparable. Politicians need money to be able to run for office. They're always under immense pressure to raise campaign funds and to be able to have those on hand, either for themselves or to help colleagues that may have a difficult race. It obviously has an impact on what we do here in Sacramento. To say that it doesn't have an impact would not be true, but it's not the only thing that drives politicians here in Sacramento.

Most politicians came up here to try and do the right thing, to try and work on behalf of their constituents or on behalf of issues that they feel passionate about. That's not true for all politicians, but it's true for the vast majority who are here to try and do the right thing.

Political Action Committee

Here at CMA, we have a PAC. We ask physicians to contribute to that PAC and we contribute to those legislators that are the most friendly to medicine.

There's nothing like somebody in the district who has developed a relationship with the legislator hosting a little event, even if it's very small dollars for the legislator. It doesn't guarantee you anything; it doesn't buy you a vote. There are no quid pro quos in this business. Anybody who tells you that's the case doesn't know what they're talking about. Votes are not for sale. You don't go around buying them.

Probably one of the perceptions about lobbyists that is the most outrageous is that we go around doing that. I don't walk around with cash in my pockets or brown paper sacks. Those days are long gone. In fact, campaign finance laws are very, very strict now, and influence peddling is a thing of another generation. So we have to be smarter in the way we work as lobbyists and that's why grassroots is very important now, having physicians get involved.

As I said earlier, nearly every legislator is up here because they are very passionate about a particular issue. That issue might not be medicine, and it might not be the thing that drives them.

Maybe education is their passion and they ran for office for because they wanted to make a change in that area. But that doesn't mean that there's not an opportunity to educate them on the issues facing medicine and affecting patient care. Since they are truly advocates for their constituents they are receptive to a message from a physician talking about what needs to be done to improve patient care.

But you also have to keep in mind that the politicians themselves are not the only decision makers. Staff is very important. We have term limits here in Sacramento, so assembly members serve for six years, Senators, eight years.

Legislative Staff Are Critical

If you're a schoolteacher or an accountant and you show up here in the state assembly, within the first year you might be chairing an important committee that has jurisdiction over health. Yet you have no health background, so they become very reliant on staff to sort through issues.

The staff have become the institutional knowledge of Sacramento, those that remember what happened two years before. But staff is very young here in Sacramento, so they're really dying and craving for information and a clear understanding of health policy from those that are actually practicing it.

Developing a relationship with those that are advising the legislators every day is very, very important. Staff should never be overlooked and they should never be dismissed, no matter how young they are.

A staff member who has responsibility for advising on health issues always looks for an opportunity to learn more about the issue. To take a tour of a physician's office, understand how patient care is delivered, how it works, how a particular specialty might be different from another is very important and very intriguing to the staff person. It is an educational process that pays off quite a bit.

Committees Require Special Attention

Physicians who live in districts of health committee members and other committees that have jurisdiction over health matters have even more responsibility to engage those legislators. All bills flow through those committees before they get to the floor of each house. A chairman or a member of a committee is going to have 20, 30, 40 votes on bills that affect medicine in as short a period of time as a month.

Those physicians who live in those districts need to engage early. They need to have breakfasts and coffees before those individuals are seeing those pieces of legislation move. We try and organize events in every district for health committee members and other committees that deal with these issues so that physicians have an opportunity to get to know their legislator better.

Face-to-face is always the most powerful, particularly if you have a pre-existing relationship with that legislator. Even if you don't, face-to-face is the most effective. Second to that is a phone call if you have a pre-existing relationship and you're able to be able to talk directly with the legislator. Third would be letters or faxes. Either one works; faxes obviously are more timely and sometimes easier to send than worrying about sending something in an envelope. E-mails are certainly the least effective along with form letters. Neither of those work particularly well.

Technology Is Changing The Process

Some legislators are starting to adapt more to new technology and pay attention more to e-mails, but at this point they're not as effective as a fax. The staff prepares a briefing packet for the legislator every day before committee hearings. Staff puts letters from constituents into the packet and they'll have a very quick briefing memo on each bill. Then the legislator is able to flip through and see the letters that were sent from the district on that issue.

Volume is critical. Most legislative offices have a multiplier effect they attribute to the letter. That is, if one person cared enough to take the time to write on the issue, that really means that there are X number of people that care about the issue in the district but didn't take the time to write a letter. So you're not just speaking on behalf of yourself, you're speaking behalf of many more constituents that didn't write a letter.

Faxes arrive on time, you can get confirmation that they are delivered and they are just as effective as sending a 'snail mail' letter. Both get opened up and the envelope gets thrown away anyway, so either a faxed letter or a regular letter will work just fine.

Start The Relationship

To best represent medicine physicians need to develop a relationship with the legislator. Very few physicians engage in politics. Part of it is just a professional distance that physicians have. Often physicians find it unbecoming or distasteful to get involved in the legislative process that is so strange to them. It is not very linear; it is not very straightforward. The best idea isn't always the idea that prevails. Politics is all about compromise and physicians often find that part of politics unbecoming.

But failure to participate lets others dictate the outcome to physicians. For decades physicians have been fighting a losing battle because they have failed to participate and because they haven't seen the value in politics. That has enabled the insurance companies and others to take a lot of power away from physicians.

Speaking For Patients

Physicians are spokespeople for patients. They have an obligation beyond just themselves to engage in the political process. Patients often struggle to find their voice; they don't have a lot of advocacy organizations here in Sacramento. It is up to physicians to make sure that patient care is the best that it can be.

So physicians need to find a way to establish relationships with legislators. They need to take the time to inform legislators on the difficulties of practicing medicine and the challenges facing not only you as a physician, but your patients as well and to be an advocate to them. When you're seen in that light, legislators will turn to you and they will seek your advice and counsel. That's invaluable.

You have to remain flexible and understand the pressures that legislators are under. Understand there are many other issues that a legislator has to deal with. At the same time they may be listening to you about healthcare, they may be hearing from people about transportation, education, the prisons, any other number of issues.

Few Physicians Are Active

I would say that less than 1% of physicians are politically active beyond just paying dues to the California Medical Association. I'm talking about taking their legislator to a lunch or to a dinner or to a breakfast.

Very few physicians take a politician to lunch, to breakfast, to coffee. When we have a physician who takes the time to establish that relationship, it's like we've struck gold. We have something that is a rare commodity. The feeling is mutual for politicians. They really seek the ability to have a relationship with physicians in their district, so when they find a physician who's willing to be active and willing to help educate them, they're very grateful.

So both us here in Sacramento on the lobby team and the politicians in the district find it helpful when a physician truly engages in the political process.

Karen S. Sealander

Karen S. Sealander is legislative counsel and lobbyist in the law firm of McDermott Will & Emery LLP, based in its Washington DC office. As a member of the Health Department of the firm, she represents healthcare providers and others on legislative, regulatory and legal matters.

Members of Congress want to hear from their constituents. They don't care what people in other districts think. They don't care what Washington lobbyists think. They care about what the people who can vote for them think. That's what sets their agenda in Washington.

Education is my number one priority. If I can educate members of Congress on an issue then we can get appropriate decisions on the issue.

You should assume that legislators know little or nothing about what you do every day, just as you probably don't know much about what they do every day.

The most effective technique is to tell them about real life examples. That real life example is most compelling. Localize your story. Tell them something that happened or might happen in your community that will affect their voters.

Those anecdotes from the district make a huge difference to members of Congress.

Another thing you can do is to invite the legislator or their staff to visit your workplace and see what you do and how it impacts their district. Invite them to come speak to your business or professional organization, especially during an election year. You can help them get good press by inviting the media to cover an event, and that's something they will value and remember.

When I go to the Hill to talk with amMember of Congress or staff and they have not heard from a constituent about the issue I want to discuss, I'm not likely to get much attention. But if I go into an office that has had the phone calls, e-mails and faxes from back home, it makes a world of difference. They sit up and take notice. They want to be helpful. They want to do what their constituents want.

Your senator or representative may not sit on the key committee that will decide the fate of your issue, but they can still influence their colleagues who are on the committees.

You don't need to know the intricacies of legislation or the legislative process. All you need to know is what you do every day. Just tell your story.

While you can have powerful influence working back home, nothing demonstrates commitment more than actually coming to Washington to meet with your legislators.

A written message to your legislators, sent by fax or e-mail to the Washington office, is also compelling. Be sure to use letterhead or otherwise include your address and contact information so that the legislator knows he is hearing from a constituent and knows where to reach you. Because of the security features in place now, using postal mail takes too long and the letters are sometimes damaged, so I advise against mailing a letter.

Numbers do count, especially if you can get lots of people to send personal, individual messages with personal stories.

Mark Cribben

Mark Cribben is the Director of FAM MED PAC for the American Academy of Family Physicians.

We're a large organization, 95,000 members. And when you go to a politician and say here's your check and by the way I have 95,000 members, people pay attention.

But for many people, for physicians particularly, politics is a dirty word, so you have to overcome the barrier of asking for the money in the first place. We explain that by pooling a lot of small donations we can make large donations to people running for Congress. That is a great advantage over individuals because they are limited to lower levels of giving. What's important is that it shows the willingness of our members to be involved politically.

PACs are the most transparent, open way of being involved. Everything we do is in the public record – the money coming in, the money going out. You don't have to pay to play. We're not buying access or influence. But you are supporting people who support your issues. It takes a lot of money to run for office. We need to be able to support the people who have helped us. They can't be elected if they can't afford to run for office.

Using Money

A PAC contribution, just like a personal contribution, gets you in to fundraising events where you can meet the candidate face-to-face. Now, you can always get an appointment and go to the member's office, but you probably won't see the member. You'll see staff. That's important and our members do that.

But at these smaller events, you spend quality time with the candidate, one-on-one; you focus on your issues. It's invaluable.

I know people worry about the ethics of using money, but members of Congress's votes are not for sale. Then the amount of money you can give, the maximum, in a two year cycle is $10,000, which is not very much when campaigns cost a million, million and a half dollars even for a small congressional seat.

Bringing in a constituent is important, probably more important than a campaign contribution. I'm on Capitol Hill every day talking to members of Congress. They see me. They know me; they know what I'm going to say. When I bring someone from the district who knows the district, particularly a physician, it's powerful.

A physician sees more voters in a district in one day than a farmer will see in a month. They know you are talking to people who can vote for them. When you come to town, it's very important for them to talk with you. Getting here to Washington and making contact are home are both extremely important.

PAC Decision Making vs. Personal Giving

You might want to give money to the member of Congress who represents you because you met them and you like them. That's great and it's not wasted, but that person may be on the transportation committee and that's not much help to our healthcare issues.

Through the PAC we are able to pool your money with other small contributions and give to someone on the energy and commerce healthcare subcommittee in the house and the finance committee in Senate. They will be handling the legislation that will affect your patients and practice.

It's important to help your local member of Congress. But as an organization, we are looking at what impacts the practice and our members. When you give to the PAC you can be sure that money will be carefully focused on our members' practice issues.

JOEL BLACKWELL 185

How The PAC Is Managed

The PAC is managed by members, a 12-person PAC Board. They are all active physicians. They approve every contribution we make. As a staff person, I work with our lobbyists to see who they are going to need to work with. I propose a list, a budget, early in the year, then the PAC board makes the final decision.

We get requests from members who aren't on the PAC board to contribute to a candidate who they think has been interested and helpful. That goes through the board as well. It's a member-driven decision with advice from us here in Washington. I love to hear from members because I can't keep track of every race in the country.

We have a candidate questionnaire we give to people who have never been in Congress. We spell out our issues, our position and ask, "What's your position?" That's a very good educational and lobbying tool, by the way, because you really have their attention.

My phone rings every day, 25 times an hour, from members of Congress, especially since we are new. We've only had a PAC for a relatively short while. Those calls are great. I use them as lobbying opportunities. It means I don't have to leave my desk to talk to a member of Congress. They are calling me. I say, "That's great, we'll consider you; and, by the way, did you know we have this issue and how do you feel about it?"

Great Opportunity

It's a great opportunity to say, "I really can't support you because this thing happened," or "I'd love to support you because you've supported us, and where will you be next week on this issue?"

It's cordial. They understand. I said no to a senator one day who called me on her cell phone and she had this event coming up and it had just occurred that she voted wrong and I had to tell her that. It's very cordial. It's an opportunity to explain why. I've never had a phone slam down on me.

Most of the time you get an offer like, come in and talk to my healthcare staff and let's see if we can work this out. It's not the money. It's that when you finally get their attention they say, "Oh, I didn't understand this issue. I want to help physicians, so let's sit down and talk."

Raising Money, For Better Or Worse

For good or for bad, they spend a lot of time on the phone dialing for dollars. They have to. Probably one full day a week they are on the phone calling people. The smart fundraisers will combine issues. For example, today is healthcare day. So they call all these healthcare groups and find out what issues they care about.

In Washington the fundraising is very business-like, very professional. You can't deliver checks in a federal building. So we go to breakfast at a restaurant or a reception. It sounds like it's glamorous and fun. It's not. It's business, particularly in the healthcare community.

Because our issues are all so related, we try to do events together. Get 10 or 12 healthcare groups around the table, all talking about two or three issues. I haven't been to too many events where you were having a great time and a few drinks. Generally you're having a muffin and coffee, if you're lucky. This is the business of politics. You have to raise funds to stay in politics and we are the people who can provide those funds.

Getting To Know You

Getting to know them is key. One thing we do in the PAC is send the check back home to a physician to present to the member of Congress. This builds our grassroots. It puts a face on the money.

We call it the three legged stool: the lobbying staff here in Washington DC, our members back home in the district and the PAC providing financial support to help candidates get elected. Those three legs support your government relations program.

An increasing aspect of our lobbying is to talk about how physicians are small businesses. They are affected by all sorts of things like any other small business – taxes, immigration, things like that.

Some small offices have one person who does nothing all day but process insurance forms. If there is some way we here in Washington can reduce that burden, it frees up resources to provide more and better care.

Personal Contributions are Also Important

It is important to write a personal check. We encourage our members to host events in their home and many do. That is the most important thing you can do. If you are willing to sponsor a party or event in your home, we will send a PAC check, a pretty big one, to such an event and then the doctors who come can write small checks as well.

To get a politician to come, the bottom line is how much you can raise. They have a limited amount of time and they have to spend it wisely; that's why the PAC will write a large check to make it worthwhile

The other thing that is valuable is the local people who come, probably leaders in the community, so it's important beyond just the money.

Recognize the Competition

We are shameless about telling our physicians what other organizations are doing, particularly those that might not have our best interest at heart. We often mention the trial lawyers. I'm an attorney myself, but now I'm on the side of the angels. The trial lawyers have been very successful raising money over the years. Physicians are late coming to the game.

What we're up against is the attorney is giving, the wife is giving, the employees are giving, all the way down the line. All perfectly legal, but everybody is giving, so they raise millions and millions of dollars.

Physicians are now coming around to the view that this (contributing money to the PAC and politicians) is a part of doing business. It's like, I pay my dues, I pay my licensing fees, I give to the PAC.

A Dollar A Day

We ask, "Is it worth a dollar a day to be able to practice medicine your way?"

If everyone in the organization gave $365 we would reach a million dollars pretty quick.

That million dollar threshold seems to be when people sit up and take notice.

We're new, so we're below 1% participation among our members. We're a big organization, 95,000 members, about 1,500 donors right now.

We think we would be successful to get 10% to give. That doesn't sound like much. I've worked with two other healthcare organizations and was able to get them up to about 30%.

Patrick F. Smith Jr. JD

Patrick F. Smith Jr. JD, is Senior Vice President for government affairs for the Washington office of Medical Group Management Association. MGMA serves 22,500 members who lead and manage more than 13,700 organizations in which almost 275,000 physicians practice.

I can communicate globally and nationally. But when a person comes in and says that Mrs. Jones needs to come in twice a week, but her insurer will only pay for once a week and as a result she can't get to the senior center, that makes a difference to a member of Congress. It personalizes it. This conveys the impact on real people.

But you don't always get to talk with a member of Congress. That's always one of the hurdles we have in the grassroots side, managing our members. They rank their experience on whether they talk with a member of Congress or a staff person. There's really no difference and more times than not, the staff person will be more familiar with the issue and more immersed in the details because they are assigned to do that.

Committee staff can be even more important. Most committee staff have been there for quite some time. They know the history. They can respond if someone asks them a question about the probability of legislation passing.

But it's not easy to see committee staff. It's more difficult for the average Joe on the street to get time with a staff member of a committee unless they are from the district of a committee member or somebody like me makes the arrangements.

Roots vs. Tops

What they are normally referred to in this town is the difference between grass roots and grass tops. They can be called on to make a contact or the member or staff will pick up the phone and call them if they have a question on a healthcare issue.

If you are running a nationwide grassroots campaign on a specific issue, you need a professional here to direct the effort. You have to have a sense from congressional staff as to why we are doing a grassroots campaign. Many times members of Congress won't be familiar with an issue and the job is to educate them. Other times they are very familiar with an issue and they aren't on your side and you are trying to influence them.

Or there are competing priorities and it's important for them to see some volume of communication so they can understand the magnitude of importance to their constituents and also to other members of Congress.

Times Are Changing

In the old days there were different hierarchies of communications based on studies of congressional staff. They would rank phone calls first, personal letters, faxes and form letters. Now we have e-mail and the mailboxes get filled up and fax numbers get changed.

The best way to communicate depends on the issue and the timing. The best way is still a personal letter or a phone call with an individual message. That's a difficult way to run a national grassroots campaign but it's critical.

You can sit in a meeting with committee staff and they will say, "This must not be important. we are not hearing from your guys." That's when you have to open the flood gates. You can do that with a scripted message you have people call or send in writing.

We have focused in the last couple of years in trying to get our members to visit their member of Congress in the home district. They are usually home Friday through Monday and we try to facilitate those meetings. You will get more time with them at home. You get a personalized, focused visit and you can do it on a weekend.

Get Politicians Into The Practice

We also encourage them to get the member of Congress or staff to spend a few hours in a practice. It's important for medical practice staff to feel it's a good business relationship, to send holiday cards, thank yous when they vote, all the relationship-building things you would do with any business relationship.

Several years ago we invested in our online advocacy center where they can send an e-mail or letter in seconds.

We can track that and over the last couple of years when we've had a big push on Medicare or something we've had 60% of our members respond. That's really high.

We believe that our members do a better job getting involved than most other groups.

Maintaining Political Neutrality

MGMA has tried to maintain political neutrality. The real strength of what we can give to Congress is our data. It's the strongest in the country and it gives us enough access. We don't need a PAC.

There's a percentage of physicians who get involved and a larger percentage who aren't. When you talk with physicians about that, they say things like, "I don't have enough time," "It's too much effort," "I'm working my tail off every day," "Politicians and the government should recognize that already," and "I shouldn't have to ask them for help."

Fact is, you do have to ask them for help. Unless you ask or tell your story about how difficult it is in the practice of medicine, they are not going to understand that there are a lot of problems.

Unless they hear from you, they are going to believe things are rosy.

The office staff is as effective as the physician in communicating as long as the communication says from the doctors clinic in

Hattiesburg and we want you to know… It's just as effective as the physician and so really doesn't take any of the physician's time.

What staff needs to understand is that they are not doing this on behalf of the physician. They are doing it on behalf of the practice for staff and patients. Staff often has the time and technological capability to communicate with members of Congress more and better than physicians.

MGMA members have a unique role in healthcare. For years when members of Congress thought about healthcare, they thought, we need to call American Medical Association. Well, healthcare is made up of clinical aspects and administrative aspects. If you don't get either of them right, you're not going to have a functioning system.

Importance Of Office Staff And Administration

In reality, more than 50% of the system is the administrative part. Our members know what's going on there.

This came home to roost a couple of years ago when there was a hearing on streamlining the administrative process and the first witness was a doctor.

He said, "Mr. Chairman, thank you for having me today. I'm really happy to be here. That's the only part of my testimony I wrote. My practice administrator wrote the rest."

When you start talking about money and contributions and employers encouraging their employees to make contributions and get into politics, people are worried that they may violate the law.

It's important for physicians to communicate and people like our guys, the head of the practice, when you are at a staff meeting or retreat to always say, "Hey, we should be talking to our members of Congress and state and local politicians."

There are no laws or prohibitions about physicians or office staff communicating   with   members   of   Congress.

Robert N. Bradshaw

Robert N. Bradshaw is executive vice president of Independent Insurance Agents of Virginia. This interview took place in his office in Richmond.

It's one thing to be aware of who your legislators are. It's another thing to be actively involved in their campaigns, serve as a treasurer for the campaign, or be politically active in the legislative efforts of members of the General Assembly. The personal relationship that our members have with their representative is something that you can't buy and you can't fake. I'm there as the hired gun to help educate representatives. But when they need examples and details, I call on the membership and they respond personally to the legislator: Here's how what you're planning to do, or establish as a law, will really work. That's something I can't bring to the table.

I would like to have as many members as possible involved in our Legislative Committee and our legislative actions.

Rank and file members can do their best by being politically active in their home town: talking to their legislators, being involved in Rotary, Kiwanis, whatever social organization that they want to be in and being good citizens.

We keep hearing about the evil insurance industry, and that's something that we really need to address. When Hurricane Isabel came through Virginia we had 425,000 claims and the Bureau of Insurance received not quite even 500 complaints on how the insurance was handled. I think that's a stunning example of an industry response to a catastrophic event, and we need to get that story out.

We try in Virginia more and more to show that our insurance industry cares about the community, the community matters. If you want to be politically active, meeting with your legislator, get active in other parts of the Association, your community, to show that the insurance industry does care, that helps just as much. But I encourage everybody to get to know who their legislator is. It's very embarrassing when we do a law and regulation class and say "who knows who their delegate is?" and only half the class raises their hands. We have to do a better job of letting people know and understand who they need to contact and when.

It's a key point that an individual may not like the insurance industry, but they certainly love their insurance agent. Legislators being human are going to be the same way. They hear all the bad press about the insurance industry. So it's our job to talk to the legislators or demonstrate to the legislators that we are actively involved in our communities, concerned about our communities and doing our best to support the communities.

We have a huge issue related to medical malpractice in Virginia, and believe me, that is not unique to our state. There are key legislators that we are going to have to meet with after the session. My goal is to get the legislators to come to an insurance office where we can meet with them or bring a couple of our members to the legislator's office where we can explore the questions they have. We need to show that we're not only people that show up during the session, but we are people that are out in the community and in their locale throughout the year.

Walking A Tightrope With Friendly Opponents

Right now we're on a tightrope between what our position is and what the doctors' position is. In some cases we're walking right down the line with them, and in some cases we're not working with the doctors. In fact they surprised us with a position on a piece of legislation this year that we thought they would support us with.

In terms of medical malpractice we want to be aware and in discussions with the medical community, but understand that we may not always agree with the medical community.

Our physicians have held White Coat Day in Richmond, which gets a lot of press. What it also does is sends legislators out to the hills, so how effective that has been in I'm not sure.

But we have to have a better understanding of what the physician communities interests are. I know the physician community has held regional meetings throughout the state, maybe we need to find a way to hold joint meetings with the physician community.

Election year is a key timeframe to meet with your legislators and talk with them.

The fact that the legislators are running for election puts them out into the community where they want to hear what their constituents are saying. So, this is a key time for our members to get out and attend political functions and listen to the legislators. They may want to ask them a question or two on how they voted on particular pieces of legislation and why they voted a particular way on pieces of legislation. Again, it's going to be incumbent upon the association to let our members know how the legislators voted. So every election cycle, it's certainly a time when the representatives go back home and hold meetings in Town Halls and go to where social groups are and speak, and that's the time to grab their ear and say there is really uncalled for legislation in some cases, and talk to the legislators.

One Powerful Volunteer Makes All The Difference

We're lucky this year that our president (a volunteer member/insurance agent) is campaign treasurer of one of the primary legislators on a major committee that oversees insurance. He has developed a long-standing relationship with this legislator. I can go into the legislator's office and say if you're not careful I'm going to set Steve on you, and he runs screaming into the night, all in fun of course.

We want you to look at who represents you and get behind that person, help them in their campaign with signs, mail, door-to-door, campaign financing, fundraising and serving as a treasurer or whatever. When these people do get elected, then the insurance agents will have that personal relationship with that individual, and that is just invaluable. You can't obtain that personal relationship in any other way.

As a lobbyist, I don't want to abuse that trust in any way shape or form. If I find it's important to call a insurance agent and say you really need to speak with your legislator about XYZ issue, that's an expenditure of trust that I don't take lightly. When I do that, it's a serious issue, and we hope that the member will contact the legislator on that, and sometimes we'll help in the visitation with the legislator. I know a lot of members, even though you feel comfortable with your legislator, you who they are, you grew up with them, when you come down to the capital, it's a scary proposition, and when you walk into that legislator's office with all the hubbub of what's going on during the session, sometimes it's nice to have a friendly person there. I like to be with our members when they go into the legislator's office.

Never Give Up Or Assume They Are Against You

Let's assume for a moment that you have a representative that just rarely supports your business interests, or they lean one way or the other in a political direction that you don't believe in. We've had occasions where we thought there is no reason for us to even go into a particular legislator's office because they rarely vote for our interests. Then we walk in and we talk to them and lo and behold they saw our position, and agreed with us. In at least two cases this year people that I would not even have suspected would be with us, turned out to be strong supporters of our position. So you really need to visit with everyone.

There is a wide range of representatives. If you don't agree with you legislator, you need to do your best to educate your legislator, and if you can't educate the legislator and you continue to disagree, then I encourage you to get active in the political campaign of their opponents. Contribute to your state political action committee, that's going to help contribute money to their opponents.

When the legislator says no, it's important to explore why the no is there. Then one of the most important things I encourage our members to do is not burn a bridge. For example, this year there was a legislator who very much supported the position that we had, but politically he just didn't think he could vote yes on a vote that was coming before us.

It was a complicated issue. This was a case when the insurance agents interests were not necessarily the insurance company interests, and he had a large company office in his district. He felt, OK, well the company frankly didn't have any votes, the agents have a lot of votes, but in this case I really don't think I can vote the way you want me to do.

No. 1, as a lobbyist my goal is to make as many people winners as possible, so this gentleman who is always, let's say 99.9% voted on our positions, I told him I would not bother him, that I would get a count of the rest of the committee. Then, if it looked like I absolutely needed his vote, then I'd come back and bother him more.

A Big Mistake You Can Avoid

Maybe he could be out of the room when the vote came up. The main thing is to not burn a bridge, not demean the legislator, continue to educate the legislator.

We have some that rarely vote in our interest. It's still important to try and educate them because you never know when they might change their minds. I've rarely run into the individual who is just going to sit there and say "I don't care what your industry says, I will always vote against you". I think if that happens you need to explore it more and maybe become politically active with the opponent.

Driving your legislator into a corner where he or she cannot win is the biggest mistake that you can make.

The representatives and senators have a wide range of constituencies they need to represent. Ninety-nine out of 100 of them do their very best to represent their constituencies, and as broad a range of their constituencies as they can. It is extremely important that you try to work and try to educate and maintain a personal relationship with your representative. Don't try to make them feel like they've lost, don't make them feel bad about a decision that they've made. It gets back to relationships with your legislator. Most important thing is, don't think you own them, I've never seen that, and it's the worst thing that you can do is walk in or call an aide and say well "they have to see me because I contributed XYZ amount of money to their campaign."

The Politicians:
How Do They Want To Be Influenced?

All politics is personal, and so are the politicians. I asked elected officials what works, how do they want to be influenced and what doesn't work.

Sen. Debbie Stabenow

U.S. Senator Debbie Stabenow of Michigan is a Democrat representing a big state. Big state senators are so busy almost no one gets to talk with them so, as she mentions, their staff have a lot of clout.

We hear from all kinds of groups, not only groups like the Homebuilders or the Realtors or the doctors, but groups of parents that come in and advocate for their children and teachers that advocate for their students. The most effective kind of message is one that comes from a personal experience.

In some way, everything gets to me, whether it is directly reading e-mail or reading a letter, or taking a phone call or whether it's a summary from my staff. On a particular piece of legislation we may get a thousand e-mails or we may get 500 phone calls on a particularly controversial issue. I'll get a summary of that, an example of the kinds of things that people shared on the phone.

Sometimes Volume Makes A Difference

Sometimes volume is important if it's a very important issue to a group of people and they have a large number of petitions or post cards, that can be something that's effective. On the other hand, sitting down with someone in their home or office or hearing their story from one of my staff about something that is unfair or unjust or a problem that needs to be fixed can be just as effective.

Story Of Dying Girl Moved Her

I have a picture on my desk of a young woman named Jessica. Jessica's mom and dad, Calvin and Tricia Luca, came to my office. They talked to me about what happened to Jessica, who is no longer living. At the time she was very ill. She had a chronic disease. Her parents had health insurance under one system and were working with a doctor who was treating Jessica. They found out they had been switched to an HMO without their knowledge. It was a complicated case.

They found out they were switched at the beginning of a month but they didn't know until a few weeks later. This was after Jessica had had an operation that was strongly recommended by her doctor but turned out not to be paid for because of this bureaucratic problem. They came to me for help and told me that working through the HMO they could not find a doctor who could treat Jessica.

In the final days of her life, instead of spending time with her and enjoying the kinds of things she loved to do, her mom and dad were spending all their time frantically dialing phone number after phone number going down a list of doctors, trying to find someone to care for her.

That was more than four years ago and that story still motivates me. I told Calvin and Tricia I would put Jessica's picture on my desk as a reminder of the need for a strong patient's bill of rights. That picture will stay there until we get it done.

In contrast, lobbyists bring the perspective of a particular group. For instance, the school board lobbyist will tell you what a particular change in the law will mean to school boards. You'll hear from the teachers' lobbyist and other administrators. You will listen to a variety of people explain what the change means to them.

But it's also important to listen to parents on issues of education, especially special education. I think the most powerful lobbying is when parents tell what the impact of a law is on them and their children. The more you can make something personal, the more effective it is.

Lobbyists And Money

There is no question that the stereotype of the lobbyist with money is very persuasive. There are six drug company lobbyists for every senator, which is astounding. But the good news about the United States of America is that in the end, each one of those lobbyists gets one vote when they walk in the voting booth. And each parent and each citizen gets one vote. And so while money is way too prevalent in all levels of government, the vote will always trump the lobbyists and the money if people are engaged and involved.

Remember that you don't always have to talk to the member of Congress. Staff are critical. I represent a state of over nine million people. I have six offices in Michigan as well as the office here in Washington.

We have 25 people here in Washington, all working in a special area, whether it's healthcare, trade, agriculture... that person is the right person to talk to if you want to find out what's happening or to make your case. That staff person is very important.

Often people think if they don't talk directly to me they aren't really getting their point across and they lose a valuable relationship with the staff. Staff are the ones following the issue day-to-day. Once you have that partnership with staff, you can be extremely effective.

It is always good to involve staff. For example, my staff goes back to Michigan on farm tours because I'm on the agriculture committee. It gives them a chance to see what's happening on the farms and in processing plants around Michigan. That's very important information.

My staffer who works on homeland security and national defense has visited Selfridge Air Force Base and local police and fire and emergency facilities. So inviting staff is important. We operate as a team and if you have a relationship with a member of the team, you can be very effective.

The most important thing is to talk person-to-person. We have a lot of issues where someone who is very liberal and someone who is very conservative work together. Right now we are working on an issue to allow pharmacists in the United States to do business with pharmacists in Canada and in other countries to bring back prescription drugs at lower prices safely. I remember working on a bill which was supported by Trent Lott who was on one end of the spectrum and Ted Kennedy on the other.

They may be supporting the bill for different reasons, but they are coming together to find a way to lower the cost of prescription drugs. This happens all the time.

It's very important not to stereotype people whether they be legislators or other groups of people. Focus on the facts and what needs to happen. Develop a strong position and try to get everybody to support it. Normally what happens is if you use common sense you can get a majority to come together.

Don Brown

Don Brown is a state representative in Florida and an insurance agent. I spoke with him as part of a project I was working on with the Florida Association of Insurance Agents.

Early in the legislative session I might not hear from too many people. But in a typical week when issues are being debated in committee or on the floor, we can get anywhere from a couple of dozen to hundreds, and I do mean in some cases more than a thousand e-mails in a week.

More than anything else, my staff and I try to separate issues based on relationships. We look at those issues that are sent to us by people we know first, and we try to give a response to everybody. I am one of the rare ones that looks at all my e-mail.

If I detect that the e-mails I am getting are form e-mails, generally I will read the first one and delete the rest. We can't respond to all of the form e-mails. If you want your e-mails to a legislator to be effective, whether it is in Tallahassee or Washington, put it in your words; don't use somebody else's form e-mail. Make it personal.

Avalanche Of E-mails

When we get flooded with e-mails, quite often it is about issues that are a statewide interest and much of that e-mail comes from outside of my district. If it is from my district it gets number one priority. If it is from the State of Florida but outside of my district, that is a second priority. Those that come from outside Florida we reserve to the end. We give priority to the people from the district first, from the state second, then if we have time, we may respond to some of the others.

If I get a constituent here to lobby and I have a paid lobbyist in my office, the lobbyist will be asked to step outside and wait until my constituent's issues are dealt with. We give far greater priority to our constituents when they come to Tallahassee than the paid lobbyist. We give the paid lobbyist our time, we give them our attention, but constituents come first.

The most important thing we need to hear from our constituents is how they believe legislation is going to affect them. What are things like in the real world? It is true that we have many opportunities to get the technical aspects of legislation explained to us by people who are very familiar with the technical and legal ramifications. What we want to hear from constituents is, "What do you believe this is going to do to you, in the way you conduct your business, and the way you conduct your life, in the real world?"

Advice For Advocates

Make contact with legislators. Let them know that you are concerned about what is going on, and begin a conversation with them. That is not where it ends, however. You need to be helpful to them. As issues come up, you need to be willing to share how you believe it will impact you.

Even beyond that, if your legislator is someone who you believe is responsive and who cares about your issues, offer to help them. Offer to help them when they run for office. Offer to help them anyway you can, to bring light upon the issues that they are going to have concerns with. You need to become their friend.

I understand the sensitive nature of this whole issue of money. But whether we feel comfortable with it or not, it is a real part of what goes on. After all, many legislators cannot afford to fund their campaigns out of their own pocket – nor should they. So being able to help with financial contributions and your time is just a part of the process. They (contributions) are just another way you can speak in Tallahassee or in Congress by helping the people who share your values, your ideas and your concerns.

Passing Legislation

The process starts with an idea. Once the idea is drafted into legislation, it is called a bill. It is introduced, quite often to several committees, and each of those committees will hear debate and they will hear public testimony. That bill very rarely makes it to the floor without change, or what we refer to as amendments.

If you know your legislator and you share your concern with them, that is not the end to it, because they have just one vote. If you have a committee with 15 members and this issue is exceedingly important to you, then it becomes very important that you extend that relationship building beyond just your legislator to all the members of that committee.

First of all, while your association has a relationship with each member of the committee and while they have the ability to communicate with them, it is quite often a smart thing for the association to contact constituents in each district of the members who sit on that committee.

Be Ready To Respond

It is important for you to be prepared to respond when your association calls upon you, so you can then place that call or make that visit to your legislator's office. Your representative may serve on multiple committees. So it is important for you to know what committees they serve on.

Know how those committees are going to take up the issues that affect you, and be prepared to share with them, not just your single self-interest, but a broader array of issues that may ultimately impact your ability to do business.

If your representative happens to be Speaker of the House, then you enjoy an advantage over many others, because in the Florida House, the Speaker of the House is a very powerful position. So you shouldn't be bashful. It is all the more reason, if you haven't already built a relationship, that you at least get to know the speaker, your representative, because when he hears his constituents, he is going to be moved by it.

One of the first things you want to do is understand that your legislator is very busy. They are going to make every effort to give you the full amount of time that you need to articulate your issue. But you need to be prepared to communicate and respond to questions – both technical questions and from a broader sense.

Your legislator may want you to be very practical about your suggestions. What is this issue going to do to you and the real world? How is it going to affect you? How is it going to affect your patients? Be respectful of their time.

What Do You Want Them To Do?

My policy is that we are going to do our best to see anybody who wants to see me. I have a personal policy that if you come to see me and my door is shut, just kick it down. But that is not the policy of everybody. They are very busy and the day can be very structured, and it helps if you will let them know in advance that you're coming. It is respectful.

Communicate what it is you want your legislator to do. Don't just complain or share your concerns. Be specific about what you want them to do. Quite often you will get a response.

Most legislators will tell you, if they understand the issue, whether or not they can support your position. If they can't, most likely they will tell you why. There are times when what you say may very well make the difference between their knowledge on the issue that gives them the comfort to be able to give you the answer.

Rarely they may tell you that they can't give you an answer. You need to be respectful for their need for additional information, but certainly don't be bashful. Ask for what you need.

If you feel strongly about an issue, even if I disagree with you, I respect your right to bring public pressure to bear upon me. But you have to be careful how you do this. Because you can get a result that you didn't count on.

Be respectful about how you go about bringing that pressure. But at the same time, this is your government. It is something that you should feel at liberty to have an effect on.

If the issue is real important and one you feel very strongly about, let your legislator know that their position is inconsistent with your position and you are going to do what you can to change their mind.

Let them know up front. Don't try to ambush them or have the media ambush them. Be upfront that you are going to communicate your displeasure with their position with your friends.

Politicians Want To Say Yes

Most legislators, me included, want to say yes. We want to please. But the time comes when we can't. It may very well be that the issue is bigger than you can realize from your perspective. After all, the scope of the issues that come before the legislature is extremely broad. The process is very dynamic.

Relationships with other legislators can be a problem. Based upon considerations beyond just the issue, it could very well be that they know that they are positioning for a more important vote coming up. They may not be able to support a bill on the committee but support it on the floor or vice versa. Inquire of them, "Why is it that you can't support my issue?" Most of them will be honest and tell you if there are other considerations.

There are occasions where leadership requests the chorus to support them on an issue. I can tell you that the higher quality of leadership, the less often they impose their will on their members.

When Leadership Calls

There are rare occasions where it is important from a procedural standpoint that we may need to get something out of committee that is not perfect so that we can posture in our dealings with the Senate. There are times when it is very important to realize that this is a team effort and you might be called upon to do some things that might not be perfectly to your liking, but you do it to be on the team.

Being a part of the leadership team is very important for your legislator. If you call upon them and insist that they do something that will destroy their relationship or impede their relationship with leadership, then you may be hurting yourself in the long run.

My advice is to be yourself. Be genuine. Make no apology for the fact that you are here because you advocate on an issue. Your legislator understands that. So don't not come and speak to your legislator out of fear that you may be perceived as being self-serving. Be genuine in your request. But make the request.

Requests In Different Forms

When the City Council or the School Board or the County Commissioners in a county that I represent pass a resolution, I pay attention. Because they are elected at the local level to represent you as well.

Quite often those resolutions may represent a narrow interest. So we have to look at the resolution and then inquire of our constituents directly if they concur with the resolution. But generally speaking, local representatives are closer than we are in Tallahassee.

I don't mean to take away from the fact that your Florida House members stand for re-election every two years; we are required by necessity to be very close to our constituents. We spend a lot of time in our district as well, but we do have a great respect for local elected representatives and we are going to give consideration to their resolutions.

Relationships Are Everything

Above everything else, in effecting the outcome of this process, personal relationships are important. In fact, if you think about it, personal relationships are important in almost anything that we do, whether it be business or whether it be dealing with our neighbors or whatever.

Following up written communications with a personal phone call, with a personal contact, being able to see a smile on someone's face, communicates more than anything in writing. So it is relationships, relationships, relationships.

But you have to be reasonable and use good manners. There are some people who have developed a talent for being a pest. However, for any legislator who is worth the salt in his bread, they will be very tolerant to a point. But when you become so persistent and go over the same thing over and over and over again, if your facts are not correct, if you are clearly off base on the issues, sometimes legislators patience may wear thin with you.

Careful Not To Push Too Hard

Most constituents don't do that, but it is a danger, and it is not different from any other relationship that you have. If you become overbearing, unreasonable or make far too many contacts – if you become the boy who cried wolf – it can make your effort ineffective.

Go back to the basics. If you do not know who your legislator is, you need to find out. Not only do you need to find out who they are, but you also need to do your own little bit of research, discover a little bit about them, find out what you can about what their special interests and pastimes are. Be able to communicate with them on a personal level.

Build A Relationship

Build a friendship and an acquaintance. It is very important that you make that effort. They have generally about 133,000 constituents in their district (state house district in Florida). They may not be able to contact each and every one individually. So there is a long line. You have to be in the line. You have to make the effort and you have to get to know them.

When you are able to contact them, be genuinely concerned about your issue, but also show an interest in the legislator. Give them information that helps them be the best they can be.

You can make a difference with one communication. It certainly helps if you can get your friends or associates to make a few contacts, because on the ordinary issues that are not high profile, 8 or 10 contacts make a strong impression on a legislator.

Know The Basics

Some people think I live in Tallahassee; others think I live in Washington DC. They are unaware that I serve in the Florida House. That is probably my fault that I haven't communicated it enough. The truth of the matter is that your legislator is in Tallahassee only a few months out of the year. Most of the year we are back in the district.

Contact Them Back Home in the District

The best place to contact the legislator is in their office in their district. You do not have to travel to Tallahassee to talk to them. If the issue is coming up in a committee, your legislator may call upon you to come to Tallahassee and testify before the committee and show your concern. So there are two aspects of visiting with your legislator.

There is certainly an appropriate time when you visit them in Tallahassee, but you can communicate your concern very powerfully where it is most convenient for you, and that is back in the district.

Most legislators would give their right arm to be able to consistently be before groups of people. Some of the legislators are better at that than others. Every time I speak to a group of people, although I have done it hundreds of times, I am nervous. But I always covet the opportunity to be able to do that. If you have a group, whether it is physicians or civic club that you could invite your legislator to speak to, they in almost every case would be most grateful.

Get Them To Visit Your Practice Or Workplace

If you can arrange for them to visit a your office back in the district, that would be very helpful. In fact if you were to arrange such a thing and be able to co-ordinate that with your legislator, that is a very effective way to get to know them and do what you ultimately want to do – to build that relationship.

There may come a time, just because of logistics or the schedule for the day, that a legislator may not be available. Most of the staff that works with legislators are extremely informed. They are very competent and capable of handling many of these issues. So don't feel bad about speaking with and sharing your concern to a staff person. That concern will be communicated to the legislator, who will follow up on that contact and be sure that your concern was adequately addressed.

Ralph Wright

In addition to a career as a schoolteacher, Ralph Wright served ten years as Speaker of the Vermont House of Representatives. When we spoke, he worked as a deputy regional representative for the U.S. secretary of education in New England. After his term as an elected official, he wrote a terrific book called "All Politics Is Personal" (1996). He was known for, and the book shows, a refreshing candor and in-your-face honesty.

His book gives a great look at the political process from inside a legislature. I liked the book so much that I talked with him about the relationship between voters and elected officials. What he says demonstrates the principles I see working all over the country.

If you were a banker in Alexandria and you wanted to influence me here in Bennington, you would a banker in Bennington. You would ask that banker if he knew Alden Graves, my neighbor. And if he said yes, then you would ask if he could get Alden Graves to deliver a message for you. Now you have to assume Alden agrees with you. What I'm saying is make it as personal as you can.

I can remember the right-to-work letters we got from all over – these pre-printed postcards – and even though they were smart enough to have people in my district sign them, I knew it was one of those automated things and people may not even have known what they were signing. If you can get somebody close to me to lean over the back fence and say, "By the way, Ralph..." that's personal and it's hard for me to say no.

I don't want to have to disappoint somebody I know, like my neighbor. I don't mind disappointing somebody who's distant.

Quite frankly, a banker would have been disappointed with me anyway because he's a banker and I'm a liberal Democrat...If I disappoint my neighbor, I have to live with him.

On some issues, they would know not to come to me if they are a bank or an insurance company. If it was something that would make the bank run more efficiently without costing anybody, sure, I would listen to them.

(Author's note: Sometime after this interview, I ran into a lobbyist from Vermont. She told me the business community got tired of Ralph's liberalism and that's why he's no longer in office.)

Most politicians will put their finger to the wind on most issues anytime they can. The problem with that is you have to constantly run the polls. Unless you have the money to do that, you never really know what your constituents are thinking. So you're always better off doing your own thinking.

Now there were certain issues I was willing to die for and I wasn't going to change. But I'm not sure all politicians find it that easy. Most kinds of issues are, "Look, if you want a bridge, I'll give you a bridge. Just put it over water. Don't get me indicted." But if you want me, in some way, to restrict the rights of my fellow human beings, you can go to hell. I'm not going to do it. Those were moral issues. I could list them on one hand.

(Author's note: There's a section in Ralph's book where he describes his battle to get a pro-choice bill passed. He tells how he got one staunch opponent, a pro-life doctor, to support his bill, which shows you should never give up on anyone.)

Even Opponents Will Help Sometimes

[State Representative] Jim Shea was a retired doctor. I had been very helpful to him, helping him campaign and in many other ways. He used my office. So I went to him and asked him for his vote on the bill, he said he couldn't do it. He was a Catholic. I got mad because he was a doctor and should understand that a woman should have a choice. I just stormed away from him. He came back the next morning and said he was wrong. What he really meant was, "I didn't want to disappoint you, Ralph. You've been so good to me."

It was very personal. Jim had lived his seventy-five years believing in pro-life, and a personal friendship changed that. He didn't want to lose me as a friend, not as the Speaker. I had been kind to Jim when kindness wasn't called for.

If you sent a crowd of bankers to me, I might be impressed by their $500 suits, but I would still resist. If you sent five hundred elderly schoolteachers, I would have great empathy. I would take time out of my day for them. Obviously I would be more likely to listen to representatives of a group than if you just walk in with no calling card. We only have so much time; the more reputable your organization, the more likely that you will get an ear. That's what lobbyists do. They represent people to politicians.

Running For Office Is A Love Affair With Voters

To a politician, when you put your name on the ballot, that's a love affair. If you lose, they don't love you.

Nobody is a step up from losing. If you're nobody, you don't know how people feel about you. When you lose an election, they have said publicly, we reject you. It's a big rejection. This ain't some girl on the phone Friday night and she says, "I'm busy," and only she knows. This is the public saying they don't love you and it's reported in the next day's newspaper for everyone to see. By the same token, it's euphoric when 51% say, 'We want you to represent us.' Then you are loved.

The Power Of Good Letters

I have received letters that motivated me to get up and do something right then.

They were all personal, hand written. If it was typed, it still had to be recognizable that the person writing this typed it; it wasn't some aide or something. They took the time, and I could read it. I would be more likely to respond to it. I would feel obligated to at least call you.

The second thing – maybe the first – is does the person live in my district? The right-to-work people who were sending me letters from all over the country…what do I care what they think in Arizona? You can't hurt me. So if you had a letter with a return address of District 1 in Bennington, I responded. I might disagree with you, but you got a response.

My secretary knew. When she opened the mail there were two piles: one was from my district, the other pile was everybody else. I had a certain time of day to read those letters. If it came from my district, I wouldn't go home without making a phone call. But you had to live in my district. You had to have some retaliatory power.

You have to get my interest. I'm a politician. If you don't get my interest, I'm going to send you a form letter. You may or may not know it's a form letter, but it's a kiss-off. You have to grab hold of me.

Power Of Lobbyists

I can insult a lobbyist and he will smile and say, "Wow, you're really funny today," because they are lobbyists. They are hired hacks. Although I like them personally, I never held them in the same esteem as somebody who lived in my district. If you lived in my district, you had a vote. If you called me, I might actually check up to see if you're a registered voter.

If you're not a registered voter, what the hell am I worrying about you for? I don't have to be polite. I don't have to put up with you haranguing me on the phone. I didn't have much patience with people who harangued anyway. But if you came from my district, I would more likely hang on the phone with you, while you were beating around the bush, to try and understand what it was you were calling me for.

Where To Start

If you are just getting started, start at the lowest common denominator, your own local representative or senator. They will listen because you live in the district. Get enough time with them so they know what you're talking about. Ask them to sit down over a cup of coffee so you can tell them about your problem. You start there.

Clay Pope

Clay Pope was a member of the Oklahoma State House of Representatives. He had previously served on the staff of a member of Congress. Thus, he brings to grassroots lobbying the view from Washington and from a state capitol. When he left the legislature he became executive director of the Oklahoma Association of Conservation Districts.

This conversation took place during a meeting of the Oklahoma Farm Bureau. I usually bring in an elected officeholder for an interview at my seminars, and this was one of the best. The points he makes about what works have been echoed across the country by federal and state elected officials.

The number one mistake people make – and I saw this both in DC and Oklahoma City – is people are very emotional. The first thing they do is kick open the door, and it's like, "You're going to do this or else."

It's just human nature that you're going to be defensive and not give as much weight to what they have to say. The other piece of that is the threat: If you don't go with us we're going to get you.

It doesn't sit well at all. Of course there are two ways to look at that. As a representative, my boss is everybody in my district.

So I want to listen to them and see what's going on. But as we all know, if you've got a boss [who], instead of coming and saying, "Hey, look, this is what we need to do…" they come in and say, "By dang this is the way it is…" that automatically turns you off.

As a legislator, I would get 40 to 50 letters a week. What I consider to be a good letter – and going back to my experience in DC as well – is something that's been written by an individual. They sit down and take the time to either type or write out by hand what their concerns are. It's well thought out. It's well put together. They're saying what they are concerned about and it's getting right to the point. That's a good letter.

I answer all the form letters too, but if somebody takes the time to really put the thought into it themselves and compose it themselves, that weighs a lot heavier on a politician's thinking, and that's generally the best kind to have.

Sometimes in Washington we'd get fifty or more letters that were exactly the same. We would write a response to it and of course [the Congressman] would sign off on it. Once it was done, we would take it and do a mass mailing.

Then whenever those form letters came in, I would give them to a woman and she automatically typed it and put their name in.

There was a place on the bottom where [the Congressman] would sign them and we'd mail them out. But basically one of those form letters was what we saw, because the rest of them were all the same.

You Must Use Form Letters

You craft one letter to cover all of those because [in Washington] you get six or seven hundred letters a week. Three times a day we'd get a stack of mail that big [shows about 10 inches with hands].

I handled agriculture, trade, natural resources and veteran's affairs, and probably every day I would get 120 to 130 pieces of mail. You just print them out automatically – the responses to the letters.

They weigh in because you keep a count of how many people were writing and how many people were sending in those messages. But it didn't carry the weight of somebody just sitting down and actually writing out their thoughts.

Petitions Aren't Worth Much

Some people bring in petitions. That's about the same as a robo [automatic mailer]. You just consider they've got one letter and they've all signed it, so you have one response to everyone who signed that petition.

When you have a petition that's got somewhere in the neighborhood of six or seven hundred signatures on it, that's the most expedient way to do it. You've responded and you've taken into consideration what they had to say. But if you had seven hundred letters that said the same thing each one a little differently, that's a lot more of an attention-getter.

People who call in, even if they all have the same basic message, it weighs in heavier than the mass mailings do because someone's taking their time and putting their dime on it. If they're making a long distance phone call to Washington, DC, or they're calling Oklahoma City, they are putting their time and money into making that phone call and you think, boy, that's somebody who feels pretty strongly about this. In my mind that's right up there underneath a personal letter.

Also you get a chance to call them back and talk to them one-on-one. You also get a chance to feel them out and see what's their thinking.

A lot of times you are looking for a solution. We don't have a monopoly on good ideas inside the legislature and in Washington, DC I mean, I'm a representative. My job is to represent, and the only way I can represent people is to know what they think. I'm their delegate in the state legislature.

There have been a lot of good ideas that have come from the district that have turned into amendments where there's been something we missed that somebody back home caught and said. "Hey, look. Did you see this? I know you guys made seventy votes yesterday. This is something I think you guys ought to take a look at when it comes back to conference committee." That really helps, and if you have a chance to talk with somebody on the telephone, I'd say that way is second behind the letters.

For every letter and telephone call I get – and this goes into the mass mailings too – I figure there are eight people at home who felt the same way and didn't call or didn't write.

Unfortunately what that does sometimes, and I saw this in DC especially, is it sets up a situation where a minority that is very well organized can drive public policy.

People From Outside my District

I get calls from people who can't vote for me and there's definitely a difference. My bosses are the people who elected me in District 59. I've got six counties in northwest Oklahoma. If somebody calls me from another town, I listen to them. But the bottom line is, my bosses are in those six counties. That's who I work for.

I appreciate anyone's input and a lot of times they've thought of something I haven't thought about. But the people in District 59 are the ones that drive the train.

That's true even when I know people have opposed me in a campaign. You may work against me. I may think you're a dirty so and so, but you're my dirty so and so and I work for you. You're the boss. I'd kind of like to have your support next time around. If I do this thing for you and I work for you, then maybe you won't be for me, but you won't necessarily be against me.

It works the other way, too. If somebody is a hard worker in your campaign, you feel a little bit more comfortable around them. I think you're a little bit more at ease and your guard is down. You say, "Okay, what can I do for you?"

It does make a difference because you feel a little bit more comfortable with them. Unfortunately, sometimes you run into a situation where you are not on the same side with someone who helped you and you just have to say, "Look, I appreciate your help. I hope it's an exception rather than the rule, but this is the way I feel about it and yes, I appreciate your support. I appreciate your help and I hope you'll be there next year, but this is just the way I've got to go and that's the way it is."

Harold Brubaker

Harold Brubaker represents Asheboro in the North Carolina House of Representatives. When Republicans were in control, he was Speaker of the House.

As Speaker I had a very large staff. I saw about one of five people who wanted to talk with me. Staff always knew to get them in if it was someone I knew.

Know the doorkeeper. If Cindy doesn't know you, you probably won't get in. You need to be able to say we've been friends for years.

The North Carolina Library Association put Richard Wells in charge of their legislative committee. He is head of the library in my hometown. I've known him for many years. The libraries got a $2 million increase in their budget, the first increase in ten years.

If you are a clerk at the 7-Eleven and I buy a drink in there every day and you call, I'll get right to the phone.

Don't write politicians outside your district. If I answer your letter, the person who represents you will come to me and ask, "What are you doing writing to people in my district?" Someone called me from Charlotte and I said, "The last time I checked, people in Charlotte don't vote in my district."

Staff is important when it comes to putting technical language in bills, but you want the elected official to instruct staff to write the bill the way you want it. You need direction from the top.

Real estate is three words: location, location, location. Politics is three words: relationship, relationship, relationship.

Cal Hobson

Cal Hobson was a state senator for Oklahoma the first time I interviewed him. I was so impressed with him that when I had the opportunity to speak with him again, I jumped at it. During this conversation he was president pro-tem of the Senate, the second or third most powerful officer in the state.

Sometime back I was scheduled to have a bill up on a Thursday afternoon. The legislature usually winds down on a Thursday and people go home. I had my votes. I was going to pass a bill. I'm on the agenda. The floor leader announces we're going to adjourn a little early. I go to him and tell him you said I could have my bill up today. And he says, it'll be just as good a bill on Monday as it is on Thursday. You'll be first up on Monday.

Okay, you do what the floor leader says. Monday I come back. The bill is in the same form, same information, and I have the same tally of votes to pass the bill. I get up and explain my bill and I lose. So I go to the back of the chamber to one of the members who had been for me on Thursday and voted against me on Monday.

"Charlie," I said, "you were for this bill on Thursday and you voted against me today. What happened?"

Overwhelmed With Opposition

He said, "Oh Cal, you just can't imagine. I was overwhelmed over the weekend with people opposed to this legislation. I had to change my vote."

So I said, "Tell me about this opposition."

"It was terrible. I got five phone calls."

He represented 30,000 people. He got five phone calls and changed his vote. Phone calls really do make a difference if done right, if you are that legislator's constituents, if you are courteous and know what you're talking about, and if you say their name

properly. Know the bill number. Know what's in the bill. Phone calls can make a big difference.

I never understood until I got there how easy it is to make a difference. I know looking at it from the outside it appears to be a complicated maze, people running around, so many bills. I'm telling you, so few people follow legislative activities, except lobbyists who are paid to be there, that it's a delight to have a real live human being walk in the door and say, "I'm here to talk to you about..."

Citizens don't do this. They don't get involved. They don't vote. They don't know who their legislator is. They don't know who their U.S. senator is, tragically enough. They don't know who is running for governor. Elected people prize the ones who do. They are informed and can make a difference in my life, not just when I'm up for election, but how I behave and think when I'm at the capitol.

Well-Informed And Involved Is Rare

You are the rarity if you are an informed, involved person wanting to talk about your profession or whatever you want to talk about. You are very rare and therefore you are very special. This (statement) is twenty-four years of experience watching it. So don't blow your chance to sit at the table and make policy.

The chair is there for you to sit in, but you have to arrive and sit in it.

The other thing that can make a difference, if you can't go in person, is a hand-written, one-page letter – not form letters or professionally organized mass mail. A real, one-page, hand-written note about the topic.

E-mail and faxes have become easier and easier. They are a little lower down on the pecking order of priority because they are easier.

Anger Doesn't Work

Don't arrive mad. Often people do. They are having to do something out of their ordinary lifestyle; they are going to a place that is foreign to them. They probably had trouble finding a place to park. If it rained, they got wet. Don't arrive mad.

Arrive with a one-page document explaining what your position is. Don't exaggerate. Tell us what is in the legislation, not what might happen if two or three years down the road such-and-such comes to pass. Legislators are thinking almost minute-to-minute. If you are talking "in three years," legislators are term-limited [in his state, Oklahoma]. A lot of them are thinking three days, not three years.

Recognize that legislator is not pulling your leg when they say, "I'm sorry, I really have to go to my committee meeting or I have to go cast a vote. I know we've only been together a few minutes." You're thinking it took me two hours to get here and this guy's only got two minutes. That's the world of the legislative session and you have to realize that and live with it.

In my state and many others, the legislature only meets for a few months. That means for seven or eight or ten months, your legislator is more accessible to you back in your community. Take that window of opportunity to get to know that person. Don't save up your thoughts for the third day of the session next year when you have your lobby day and everyone comes to the capitol.

Offer to buy coffee or lunch, if that's permitted, and it's not in some places. Speak to them in the post office. You are miles ahead. You are already at the table because you know them. It doesn't have to be intrusive. It doesn't mean drop by unannounced.

If the legislator is in their favorite coffee shop having breakfast, it's fine to ease over and say, "Hi, I live in your district and I'm a dental technician. We've got an issue coming up I'd like to talk about sometime when it's convenient; here's my card. Could you give me a call when you have time?"

What's not cool is to plop down in the booth and wax eloquently about your cause for an hour. You wouldn't want it done to you and legislators don't want it done to them.

Politicians Are Human

It's amazingly not realized that politicians are human. We are the focus of so much of the evening news, good and bad. We appear to be so distant. Many people when they think about politicians think exclusively about Washington.

I can't tell you the number of times people have said to me, "I'm upset about the Department of Defense or the CIA or Russia." We don't deal with those issues. We are not Congressmen. We are state legislators. You need to differentiate.

It does appear to many people that we are a distant class, almost a ruling class. That leads to anger, frustration and dropping out, which is the biggest mistake people can make. If you are not in the arena early and often, I assure you, everybody else is. Then their issue is heard and dealt with, and yours is not.

Contributing money helps. There's not a darn thing wrong with helping candidates who agree with you have the resources to win. In all likelihood, for every issue that you are an advocate for, there are people on the other side and they are funding candidates they agree with.

In Oklahoma the maximum you can give is $5,000. I know that sounds like a lot of money. It is a lot of money. But any politician that would sell a vote for $5,000, (1) is crooked (2), will get caught (3), will go to jail...so why even think about doing it?

What Money Doesn't Buy

So if you are giving a check thinking I now have bought Senator X or Representative Y with my check, erase that thought from your mind. All you're doing is saying, "I understand it takes money to run for political office. I want to help you be successful."

Down the road, lobbyist organization XYZ is going to come to the capitol and may even say, "Remember, I helped you last summer. Remember me, I knocked doors for you." That legislator better remember that. That's okay.

What's not okay is to go the next step. "Because I maxed out to you with my contribution of $5,000, you are going to vote for Senate Bill 24 or I'm never going to help you or vote for you again." That conversation cannot be had. That suggests the money was given as a future bribe to buy votes. Don't go there. Don't do that.

Back when deregulation of electricity was a big issue, California had passed deregulation and we all saw what happened with shortages and high prices. An environmental group, Sierra Club types, came to me back home in Norman. This was after I had voted for Oklahoma's version of deregulation.

They said, "Look, Cal, you see the consequences of this. Here are documents to confirm what we are telling you." And so I had a fundamentally different view of the risk that issue had for our state. It was because of a very energetic advocacy of people on the other side that I respect and trust.

Sometimes you have to say no to people, people you like. To be honest, it's very painful at the moment. Especially if it's important.

There are lots of bills that aren't important. But if you vote against a lobbyist that you like – some of them you like a lot, some you like a little and some you don't like at all – when you have to look at a friend – a lobbyist you've known for twenty years and you know it's almost his life is on the line, or at least his economic life is on the line, or his success with his group – and you have to tell him you just can't vote with him, it's very hard.

Letting Down Your Friends

At the end of the day, after you've cast sixty votes, maybe more, you've got to go home, not beat your wife, not abuse the children. Just recognize that from their point of view, you let some friends down that day because you couldn't vote with them.

You have to get up the next day and go back into that environment and you are hoping there will be another day you can help the group you couldn't help before – not as a payback, simply as a reality of how the democratic system works. It makes you feel better when you can do that. Hopefully the lobbyist and their group will say, "Well, ol' Cal blew it three weeks ago, but he got this one right."

It's human nature. I'd be a big fibber if I said everybody who comes through the door is exactly equal and they are all going to get the same response. That's just not true. We are all human. People I've known for many years, who've never deceived me, who've always given me the truth, they probably get a break.

If a group has been with you through many tough battles, in my case, educators, you tend to not ask as many questions, to recognize where the battle line is and come to the conclusion, yes, I can do that. There may even be some short-term pain. Sometimes you are voting because of that personal relationship and commitment when it's a close question.

Mail From Outside The District

A lot of members throw mail away or don't return phone calls if they come from outside the district. You have to know where to target. If you have a water issue in southeast Oklahoma and you're bugging the guy in the panhandle about the water issue, you're talking apples and oranges and he's not interested. You have to know how the issue plays in that member's district. Then you have to lobby him not top down, but bottom up, where the voters are.

Role Of The Lobbyist

People forget this or don't know it. They think their lobbyist can do it all. It's okay to be well represented by lobbyists at the capitol. It's more than okay; it's crucial. You can't succeed at the state capitol without effective representation.

But that only takes the ball part of the way down field. On a tough issue if the legislator is not hearing from people back home, the lobbyist is just one voice. If it's a tough vote, a tax vote or an environmental vote, you must have your message coming at that senator or representative from both directions, the professional information and data swirling around the rotunda, and he's also got to hear from back home why it's important and why we're going to tilt him to do something that's tough.

No Vote Is Always Easiest

Remember in politics, the easiest vote is always no. You can always say, "I didn't know enough about the issue. Nobody had talked to me about it." You can wrap yourself in the flag of ignorance. If you vote yes, that means change.

That means consequences for you as an elected official that do not arise from a no vote.

If you want something proactive, that's always harder. Status quo is easy. Getting a yes is doubly hard, and if you don't have help from back home, you're fighting with one arm behind your back and you're more likely to lose.

Congresswoman Linda Sanchez

Congresswoman Linda Sanchez represents the 39th District in California, which includes part of Los Angeles. Sanchez's service is historic as she joins her sister Loretta (D–Garden Grove) in the U.S. House. They are the first sisters and the first women of any relation ever to serve in Congress.

We get all kinds of lobbyists coming in. They typically know their issues, but they can't give the perspective that an individual member of an organization can.

I have lots of groups and individuals come in to talk. If you are going in to talk with a member of Congress about an issue, be specific about what you want them to do. Get that out in the first five minutes of the conversation. That's the best thing you can do.

I have had folks come in and spend the whole meeting time talking about the history of the organization, how they came into being. Often we already know that information. We're looking for what you want to talk about. Get that out in the first five minutes so the majority of the conversation can be about what concerns you.

We have had people come in, they start off with small talk, they give me the history, how many members they have and they'll leave the office and I won't even know why they came in to talk or what they were concerned about. That's not really an effective way to use the limited time you are going to have with members of Congress.

We are very committed to serving our constituents. Regardless of party affiliation, our job is to work with all the people from our district. I meet with people of both parties or third parties or independents. It has very little bearing on the issues we talk about. I don't have preconceived ideas that this person is from that party so I'm not going to listen to them. I'll meet with anyone from the district that we can work into the schedule. Often we don't see eye-to-eye.

But I'm respectful enough to anyone who takes the time and trouble to make an appointment to come and see me to give them a chance at least to express their point of view.

We may have a back-and-forth dialog, I may change my opinion; I may not. By virtue of the fact that I always respect people who come in, I always expect people that I don't agree with to respect my point of view. You can have a discussion of differing points of view as long a people agree to respect each other.

One of the things I like to do is go back to the district and tour a facility that employs people. I recently did a site visit to a plant that made the toolboxes the municipal trucks. They didn't have enough space to park the completed vehicles before the moved them out to the dealerships or owners.

There were some adjacent pieces of land owned by Southern California Edison that had utility lines over them but space on them where the trucks could be parked. I was able to work with the company and southern California Edison so they could rent the land to park the trucks. That is something I probably never would have known about if I hadn't gone on that tour. Site visits are very helpful to understand the problems businesses have.

We can't meet with everyone, so often we rely on our staff. People who don't get to meet with a member shouldn't take it as a sign of disrespect. Meetings with staff are the next best thing. Usually I will get a memo if not an oral briefing about what issues came up. It's not as effective as a meeting with the member, but it's the next best thing.

If you are meeting with staff out in the hallway, maybe there's something implied in that. But if you're meeting in the office they are doing their job and they will be advising the member.

Staff:
Influential, And Key To Your Success

Legislative staff whether in Washington DC or your state capital is just as important, sometimes more important, than the politicians. Their recommendation is often the final decision.

Many of your political interactions will be with staff members, some of whom may be quite young and have a different outlook than yours. More and more, I am advising clients to think about selecting at least one person for the contact team who is a person of color and/or female and/or in their twenties. I try to avoid using groups of white, middle-age men in pinstripe suits, since people on the Hill are diverse and sensitive to issues of diversity.

State legislators tend to have no staff or just a part-timer, so you can usually get to a state senator or representative directly. Committee chairs at the state level may have staff they will want you to talk with. All staff are important. They can put your call through or put you on hold. They can report your message with enthusiasm and advocacy, or negatively.

Court and cultivate all staff just as you would a politician. Common titles and roles in Congress include the following:

Administrative assistant (often referred to as the AA or chief of staff). Reports directly to the elected official. May have overall responsibility for evaluating the political outcome of legislative proposals and constituent requests. Usually in charge of office operations, including the assignment of work and the supervision of key staff.

Legislative assistant (LA) or legislative director (LD). Monitors legislative schedule and makes recommendations regarding issues. Some offices, for example in the U.S. Senate, will have several LAs focused on narrow policy areas such as taxation, healthcare, the environment, and so on. This person may be the last one to speak to the official about an issue prior to a vote or decision. They carry a lot of weight and have a lot of power.

Press secretary, communications director. Often has multifaceted role of ensuring constructive flow of information between the elected official, the media, constituents and public. Will be especially sensitive to any media lobbying techniques.

Appointments secretary, scheduler. Allocates official's time. May be responsible for travel arrangements, speaking engagements and coordinating work in the district. This person's primary job may be to protect the elected official's time from people like you.

Case worker. Helps constituents deal with bureaucracy. Prepares communications with agencies and to constituents.

Below you can see the kinds of salaries staffers make and get an idea of how various offices are staffed. You won't find all these titles and people in every office, since every office is different. The senior people, if they choose, can usually find a job in the private sector making three or four times these salaries. There is a lot of turnover and there are a lot of people in their early and mid-twenties, many in their first job. Many move on to become professional lobbyists.

U.S. Senate staffs vary, depending on the population of the state.

Approximate Salaries of Congressional Office Staff
Committee staff salaries are generally higher

Chief of Staff	$117,000
Legislative Director	$ 92,000
Deputy Chief of Staff	$ 88,000
Communications Director	$ 65,000
Legislative Counsel	$ 60,000
Office Manager	$ 58,000
Personal Assistant	$ 50,000
Legislative Assistant	$ 45,000
Scheduler	$ 44,000
Project Manager	$ 44,000
Constituent Services Rep	$ 41,000
Systems Administrator	$ 40,000
Correspondence Manager	$ 36,000
Assistant to the Chief of Staff	$ 32,000
Deputy Communications Dir	$ 31,000
Computer Operator	$ 29,000
Research Assistant	$ 28,500
Legislative Correspondent	$ 25,000
Correspondence Assistant	$ 23,100
Staff Assistant	$ 22,504
State Office Staff Director	$ 74,000
Regional Manager	$ 40,500
Office Manager	$ 37,500
Scheduler	$ 34,000
Constituent Services Representative	$ 30,000
Staff Assistant	$ 24,456

This staffer for a member of the U.S. House did not want to be identified for obvious reasons. I asked him what he does with the information left by all the people who come in lobbying.

At the end of the day, we tell him [the member] who came in and what they wanted. If I don't know for sure he knows them, or it doesn't seem important, I don't mention it. He sees the list and sometimes will ask who people are, sometimes not. He trusts me to let him know if he needs to know.

Lots of people come in to blow off steam or get a hearing. If we listen, they're happy.

Nicole Rutberg

At the time of this conversation, Nicole Rutberg was the legislative assistant for Senator Charles Schumer (D-NY). Like all senators from the large states, he is crushed with people wanting to see him, and so is his staff. Only a small percentage of people get a personal conversation with U.S. senators from large states like New York, Florida, or California, so it's especially important to work with their staff.

Many times when a group comes in, it will be me and a group of older men. I look very young and sometimes I can see in their faces that they wonder if I am the appropriate person for them to talk to. It takes a few minutes for them to adjust and realize they need to deal with me. If I bring in another person, they need to give us equal attention and not decide on their own to focus on the other person.

People come to see me on a minute-by-minute basis. I get about twenty voice mails an hour. One day our office got 925 calls; the average is eight to nine hundred. When I'm out, I'm afraid to go back and check my messages.

People need to remember that staff is very transient. The person you talked to before may not be working in that office or may not be handling your issue any more. Call and ask who is handling your issue. Each staffer handles about ten issues. Several people may be handling an issue and you need to coordinate with all of them. For example, three people in our office handle transportation issues.

Most appointments will be for thirty minutes. Plan your presentation for twenty minutes or less because we want question time. We have so many meetings; unless you have something new to say, don't schedule another meeting. It takes away from time that I can be doing your work.

When things are in the media, it gets our attention. That's one way staff finds out what is going on. When issues are in the media it gets the attention of local, state, and federal leaders.

Jim Brandell

Jim Brandell was chief of staff for U.S. Representative Dave Camp, member of the Ways and Means Committee, when I spoke with him.

The volume of communications we get is tremendous and growing all the time. It's probably doubled in the last four years because of technology. We probably get over 3,000 constituent letters a month that need to be responded to in some way.

Since the anthrax scare and 9/11, regular mail is severely delayed. It can be two or three weeks, sometimes more than a month delayed. We encourage people to either fax or e-mail to our office.

We get about a thousand scheduling requests every month. Someone who is asking for the Congressman's time or to come to a reception. A lot of it is generic – they invite everybody in Congress – but they still have to be looked at.

(Author's note: I should probably write a separate section on receptions, since this is a common way to meet with members of Congress. Suffice it say that one day in Washington I went to a reception on Capitol Hill with some clients. The caterer told me there were twenty-four receptions going on that day that he knew about.)

We have to prioritize. Who is asking for the meeting? Is it someone from our district? Or is it someone who has an interest in our district? Do they have an issue that is before the Congressman's committee? If you have an interest before his committee and an interest in Michigan, you're probably going to see the Congressman personally, at least for fifteen minutes.

He's very constituent oriented. Most members of Congress are. If something has a direct impact on the district, that's very important. If it's more general to Michigan or it's a group he's seen several times before, or there aren't any constituents, he may have a legislative assistant meet with them, especially if there are hearings going on and he needs to be there. On Ways and Means there are hearings going on all the time.

On a typical day in March and April, when most associations come to Washington, the Congressman might have ten to fifteen different meetings in fifteen-minute increments. We have four different legislative aides and a legislative director and they might have ten- to fifteen-meetings a day in a busy week.

If it's a constituent, or if it's an association or someone who works with us, like Denise (the lobbyist for the association hosting the meeting) who wrote us a letter, she's not a constituent, but she's from an association we work closely with, and that gets bumped up to the legislative aide.

We have a three-day turnaround on all our mail. If someone writes a general letter on an issue and is not a constituent, we'll probably refer that letter to the appropriate Congressman.

Not A Constituent, No Answer

Just because of the sheer volume, we can't answer pieces of mail from people who are not from our district and are not from an association that we have a relationship with.

Every week we put a report together for the Congressman of our top twenty issues so he sees what people are writing about. Congressman Camp, and this is not true of all members of Congress, personally signs all the letters that go out of the office. He may not read each letter individually, but he will see that Jane Doe from Saginaw is writing him and if he recognizes the name he'll look to see what the issue is.

People Who Are Known Get Attention

I look at all the letters before they go out. If there are certain issues that are hot, we bring a sample of letters to him. If there is someone he's known over the years, someone we've been working on an issue with, we bring that to him. We have legislative meetings with him twice a week where we go over issues and bills and we bring up letters then as well.

Even if it is a generic letter, the exact same letter from two different people, we still respond. We might send a standard response, a thought-out response. But if there is something personal there, "I saw you at the Kiwanis or I appreciated your comments at the Kiwanis," you're going to get a different response. Making your letter personal definitely makes a difference.

Congressman Camp represents fourteen different counties, so we have a variety of media to watch, several radio stations and TV stations and so forth. We subscribe to all the newspapers, the ones that aren't online. We clip and scan the main stories that have federal implications. Every two days he gets a packet of clips. Our staff back in the district monitors print publications. Our communications director monitors the online ones. There are some great services that monitor issues we want to keep informed about and they send us packets as well as anything his name appears in.

Working With Staff

You have to realize that 25-year-old legislative assistant has been working night and day on the issues you are talking about. She's been sitting for hours in committee meetings hearing professionals testify, reading Congressional Research reports about the issue, writing very thoughtful letters back to individuals. She's usually very well briefed on your issue. Don't let the age fool you.

These jobs are incredibly demanding and so the younger people tend to take these jobs.

I am the oldest person on the staff. I'm thirty-six.

Mistakes People Make

It's hard to characterize anything as a "mistake." Just by coming in, they've done a good thing for democracy and for their issue. It's great when people do that and I wish more people did. I think people forget how accessible government is. They have this feeling that Washington is an arm's length away and I can't get anything from my representative.

When someone comes in as a volunteer advocate, they need to remember where we're coming from. We have ten issues just from Ways and Means Committee let alone the whole Congress we're dealing with. They need to be concise. Are they here to advocate for a bill? What's the bill number? Why are you here? Why is it important to you? What implications does it have for the Congressman in his home district?

You don't have to know everything. Just the basics. Boom. Boom. Boom.

A lot of times they come in not being very specific, not being conscious of the time constraints of the Congressman or the staff, and then forgetting what the follow-up needs to be. What's the ask? Make sure you don't forget the ask. You want him to support a bill? You want him to sign a delegation letter?

We want to see people from our district; otherwise they're not going to meet with the Congressman. They need a personal anecdote or something to help us understand why it's important to them. We know the policy stuff from the professional lobbyist and professional staff. The importance of the volunteer is to add a different dimension, a real-life scenario of how this impacts them in the Congressman's district.

Get The Card For Follow-up

Before you leave make sure you get the card of the aide you talked with. Ask if it's all right to follow up with you. Is e-mail the best way? Or a phone call? They'll probably say e-mail is best way because of time constraints.

Make sure you know whom to follow up with and at what time. Could I follow up in two weeks to see if you cosponsored the bill? Could I follow up in a month? What's a good time frame given the legislative calendar?

We have two offices in the district. It's fourteen counties, one of the largest congressional districts. Our district operation focuses mainly on casework, whether that's immigration, Medicare, Social Security, military issues.

Back Home In The District

The staff there works to help people deal with government agencies to help people get help and answers. That's their main focus. There's someone there I work with closely on the Congressman's district schedule. Our legislative staff and communications staff and the main scheduling staff are here in Washington.

I go back to Michigan to meet with the district staff at least once a month.

We have weekly meetings where the district staff is conferenced in by phone so they know the hot issues. They get a lot of phone calls like, vote no on this bill coming up, so we make sure they are briefed on what's coming up. They have their specific duties with regard to casework, but we have to be in close contact just because a constituent doesn't care if they call the district office or the Washington office, they want an answer.

He's very interested in doing site visits, plant visits, things like that. He likes to have a staff member go first to see the facility, almost like an advance visit. If you invite him, our district director would probably go take a short tour. He would probably report back this is a great facility and the Congressman really needs to stop by here.

Mentioning Contributions

If you've met the Congressman at a fund-raiser, you can bring that up. "Oh, it was great seeing you at breakfast the other day; now here's the issue we want to talk about." There's no problem with that, but I wouldn't bring up a dollar amount, as in, "We gave you a thousand dollars last year and you didn't support us." That wouldn't be the way to go.

If you are trying to develop an advocacy network, it's important to develop that relationship ahead of time. Then find out who in the office handles the issue you are concerned about. Ask for their e-mail and drop them a note. If that person is familiar with you, they will give you more attention when things come up.

When you come to meet with a Congressman or staff, they are there to listen to you about what's important to you. They want to know what concerns you have and what's personal to you. Just know what point you want to make, that's the main thing. Don't worry about last year's legislation. If you don't know something, just say let me have our association staff follow up on that.

Find Local Campaign Events You Can Attend

My boss has several events going on during the year. We have a family picnic where you can go for $45 and take the whole family. Start with something like that. Introduce yourself. Most members of Congress have things like that – low dollar events you can go to. You can often meet staff members there as well.

Obviously the national association is going to contribute at a higher level, but you can find some low-dollar events where you can make a face-to-face contact with the Congressman. That's a great way to start.

We deal with a huge variety of issues. So you need to excuse us if sometimes we seem aloof, like we're don't know what you're talking about when you walk in the door. We might have just got out of a meeting on textile imports from China. If we seem short or in a hurry it doesn't mean we're not interested. Don't assume we are completely up to speed. Brief us on the basics for a minute or two. The Congressman would definitely appreciate that if you meet with him personally. He's just taken a school group on a tour of the capitol and has been in a committee meeting so he needs to be brought in, here's the issue, here's what it's about. Be concise.

Make The Ask

Ask for what you want. You have no idea how many times people have a meeting, talk about something, and forget to do ask or forget to find out where the proper follow-up channels are. It helps us to have a specific ask and set time frames for response.

It's best not to overcrowd the meeting. We've had groups of twenty people. That's too many. The offices on Capitol Hill are pretty small. Most offices don't have a conference room. Usually the legislative staff is going to meet with you right in the lobby where you walk in. Or they're going to take you out into the hall where there's more room. It's no slight to you; we just don't have the space.

If you're meeting with the Congressman, you can go in his office and shut the door. Upward of five people would be the most that would be reasonable. I wouldn't bring more than five.

Make sure you have your business cards there to hand out and be sure you follow up. Once a week would probably be too much. Twice a month would be sufficient in most cases if it's a short communication.

Sarah Dufendach

Sarah Dufendach was administrative assistant to Rep. David Bonior at the time of our conversation. Later she was Chief of Legislative Affairs for Common Cause, the citizens advocacy group.

Rep. Bonier sees a lot of communications from constituents. Especially if someone takes the time to hand-write a note, he sees that stuff. Also, we keep a real good tally of who calls on what issue, are they pro or con, how passionately people feel when they call, who's in the district, who's out of the district. He gets a report on that twice a week from the receptionist who takes the calls.

He always wants to know how are the calls running, how is the mail running, what do people in the district think about what is going on.

What Does He Want To See Personally?

The kind of letter that he would take a look at is one that is particularly representative of what people are thinking. If we get fifty letters coming in and they all say pretty much the same thing, one of those would get to him. If it's handwritten or it's a personal story, those kinds of things he loves to read.

When we were going through the NAFTA debate, there were some strawberries that got contaminated with pesticides. The mother of one of the little girls who got sick sent a letter. While we were already inclined to be on her side, her letter was so compelling she energized us to do even more about food safety and labeling. She motivated us in a very personal way.

The kind of thing he looks for that's different from a lobbyist is a personal story, a personal circumstance – something where a piece of legislation would affect somebody's life. Sometimes lobbyists can put things in terms that are very canned, very perfect. We don't look for perfect.

We would rather have somebody write on a paper bag about something that is real to them than on a nice flashy glossy piece of stationery from a lobbyist downtown because that may or may not be real. But if somebody takes the time to call or include a personal story or a picture of themselves, that lets us know they really care and we will care in kind.

Don't worry if you don't get to talk with the Congressman. Sometimes people will come here and the staff they meet with are barely old enough to be their children. You have to remember, it's a real sacrifice for work in government on the hill. The pay isn't good. The working environment is crowded. The hours are long. Most people here have a real sense of purpose. They want to do the right thing. They want to learn. They want to learn from the people that come to them. Even though they are young they are very dedicated. They are the best and brightest. It's incredible the talent we get.

If you try not to figure out how young they are, you might learn something. The young person who looks like they just had purple hair yesterday is the person who is in position to take the tally notes. Very often the receptionist keeps the member's schedule and can help you get in or not get in. It can be very deceiving that people who look like they don't have any power do have a lot of power.

Be An Effective Grassroots Lobbyist

Don't feel everything you say to us has to be perfect. We see perfect a lot from people in town and we don't need that. It does need to be real – a story you have lived in your daily life. If the river is polluted and you can't run your boat, that's something you can tell us. It's going to be a river we know, a marina we are familiar with.

Just come in and tell your story the way you see it. Don't be afraid. You don't have to worry about dressing right or knowing everything about a piece of legislation. You don't need to know the vernacular. It doesn't matter. It's refreshing when people don't know H.R. this or that.

It's great for people to come to Washington. It's an absolutely beautiful city. It's filled with all the lore and history of our American heritage. Also, you see that we are people just like you. We have kids. We have problems. We know what you're feeling, the grocery prices. Sometimes it's reassuring when you can just talk to a human being.

The importance of having a meeting one-on-one is like any other human interaction. It's easier when you can put a name and a face together. It's easier to communicate if I can see you. I can watch your expressions. I can ask questions. I can elicit responses. You get a feel for what's going on.

Paul Reagan

Paul Reagan was administrative assistant to U.S. Representative Jim Moran (D-VA). He had worked for four members of Congress.

You want to show members that this is truly a grassroots campaign. You want to create the impression of a groundswell of public opinion. It's the quality of communication rather than the quantity that counts. This week we are getting a bunch of letters on an environmental issue. They're all identical. It has a far smaller impact.

When the letters are individual and show how it impacts people and their business, it has much greater impact.

Never threaten. Don't link anything to money [contributions]. You will lose credibility and respect.

Use the press in a positive way. Don't buy paid media ads that mention elected officeholders by name. They just feel threatened. One of the best ways is to get local editors to write editorials. Letters to the editor have great impact.

People on the hill are very busy. It's important to follow up. Sometimes things get dropped or fall through the cracks.

Getting To Be Systematic
And Deliberate

You can have enormous political power.

The system is outlined in this book. What I have described is nothing more than a compilation of tactics, techniques and strategies that work.

But you must make a deliberate decision to use this system.

I cannot promise you will win everything you want. You probably will suffer disappointment like Dr. Glomb. But I can promise if you do not get engaged, you will get nothing, and may have something taken away.

If you follow my suggestions, persist no matter what and keep a smile on your face, you will almost certainly win something.